Penguin Health

How to Lose Weight Withou

Michael Spira was born in 194— — — —owe School, and qualified at St Bartholomew's Hospital, London. He has written several books and many articles on health and medical topics, and he has made several radio broadcasts and television appearances. He has lectured widely on the subject of obesity and slimming.

He is married and has two children, Tiffani and Robin. His interests include music, cricket and good food (slimmers please note!).

Michael Spira

How to Lose Weight
Without Really Dieting

Penguin Books

PENGUIN BOOKS

Published by the Penguin Group
27 Wrights Lane, London W8 5TZ, England
Viking Penguin Inc., 40 West 23rd Street, New York, New York 10010, USA
Penguin Books Australia Ltd, Ringwood, Victoria, Australia
Penguin Books Canada Ltd, 2801 John Street, Markham, Ontario, Canada L3R 1B4
Penguin Books (NZ) Ltd, 182–190 Wairau Road, Auckland 10, New Zealand

Penguin Books Ltd, Registered Offices: Harmondsworth, Middlesex, England

First published by Penguin Books 1978
Reprinted 1979
Revised edition 1988

Copyright © Michael Spira, 1978, 1988
All rights reserved

Set in Plantin and Rockwell by
Rowland Phototypesetting Ltd,
Bury St Edmunds, Suffolk
Made and printed in Great Britain by
Cox & Wyman Ltd, Reading, Berks

Except in the United States of America, this book is sold subject to
the condition that it shall not, by way of trade or otherwise, be lent,
re-sold, hired out, or otherwise circulated without the publisher's
prior consent in any form of binding or cover other than that in
which it is published and without a similar condition including this
condition being imposed on the subsequent purchaser

Contents

Preface to the Revised Edition

The first edition of this book was looked upon as something of a revelation because no one had previously written a 'no diet' slimming book. The book appealed to many people who found that it helped them to lose weight painlessly and permanently.

But since that first edition I have found that some slimmers need more detailed advice about the psychological aspects of slimming. I have gradually devised a series of eating 'hints' which almost every slimmer will find useful, and these are incorporated in this new edition.

Another new feature is the inclusion of one week's menus. These illustrate further some of the calorie-saving principles described in this book and they also demonstrate that your food can be both economical (in terms of calories) *and* delicious.

Happy slimming!

Acknowledgements

I owe an immeasurable debt to my wife, Alison, both for her encouragement and for her written contributions. In particular, the recipes in this book I owe entirely to her.

Introduction

Why add another book on slimming to the dozens already available? Before fully answering this question it is worth mentioning that most doctors find that the problems connected with being overweight concern many people. With the increasing public awareness of matters of health, more and more people are realizing that they are overweight, and more of them are trying to do something about it. The problem is that such a large number of people fail in their attempts. Or, if they have managed to lose weight, many of them fail to keep to their new weight. But this is hardly surprising when one considers how many of them rely on slimming tablets, slimming aids, counting calories or carbohydrate units, or slavish adherence to diets. These methods do not encourage permanent sensible eating habits and often demand too great an element of will-power, a mathematical mind capable of juggling with lots of figures, or assume that everyone walks around with a set of pocket kitchen scales and pocket calculator.

This book contains the secret of successful slimming. No pills, no diet sheets, and no need for any kind of medical supervision – just the simplest, and oldest, way ever devised to lose weight, as successful slimmers will know. It is the most logical way – just eating less. But, and this is the important point, *only a little less*. Two potatoes instead of three, one slice of toast instead of two – just that *little* bit less that is barely noticeable. Apart from a few modifications which are described in this book, the food you eat need be no different from that which you have always enjoyed. And new eating habits become a permanent way of eating.

But if the method is so simple why is there the need for a book about it? There are two reasons. First, because the method is so simple people often view it with scepticism until they are shown with figures some of the ways, many of which may not be so obvious, that calories can be saved. In addition, there are a number of hints and psychological 'tricks' which are enormously useful. It is rather like a motorist being told that the secret of saving petrol is to use less of it. But *how* do you use less? After all, the accelerator, the choke, the gears, the clutch and the brakes all have to be involved. So what is the relative importance of each? A motorist who has been shown the many little driving techniques will get far more mileage out of each gallon than the motorist who has been given only vague advice such as 'use less throttle'.

The analogy of the motorist lends itself to the second reason for this book. To achieve success a motorist needs not only to know how his car uses petrol, and why the techniques he has been shown work, but also a rudimentary knowledge of how to keep his car in good working order. Similarly, in order for the slimmer to apply successfully an idea which is so simple, flexible and adaptable, it is important to understand the medical significance of being over-weight and the principles of sensible nutrition and physical fitness. For this reason topics not directly related to slimming such as cholesterol, dietary fibre, exercise and so forth are included.

Although it is impossible to answer or anticipate all the questions that a would-be slimmer might ask, I hope that this book will answer most of the questions, such as why people become overweight, and why slimming tablets are not the solution to weight problems. Other topics include the problems of childhood obesity.

Fortified with this knowledge I feel that the reader will appreciate and more readily understand – and perhaps be more motivated towards – the slimming principles described in this book.

1

Am I overweight?

The chances are that you are overweight for that is probably why you are reading this book. But, you may ask yourself, how do I *know* that I am overweight? I may look overweight, and people tell me that I am fat. But surely that does not necessarily prove that I am overweight.

Already you have almost answered your own question. You look overweight and you look fat. *How* you look is one of the best indications as to whether or not you are overweight. If you look in the mirror and you see a fat person, then that person – yourself – is overweight. And immediately you have found the key to what being overweight is. Too much fat. Your body is carrying more fat than it needs.

But why does the body need fat at all? How unkind of nature to invent something that most of us spend a good deal of our lives trying to get rid of. The answer may seem surprising, but the simple fact is that fat is an organ of the body.

Organs are tissues composed of cells that are grouped together into structures which have specific functions. The most familiar organ to most people is the heart. Its function is to pump blood around the body in order to provide oxygen to the tissues and to remove the waste matter which is produced by the body's chemistry. The lungs are the organs with which we breathe. The kidneys remove many of the waste products of the body by excreting urine through yet another organ, the bladder. Similarly, fat has a definite role. It provides the body with a layer of insulation, helping to keep the cold out and to retain the body's heat. It is also an important source of energy for the body, and this is described in Chapter 4.

Fat is therefore necessary for the body. But our bodies need only a certain amount of it. It is when too much fat is present that we become overweight.

But just because I *look* overweight, does it mean that I necessarily *am* overweight? I may look big because I have large bones. Or I may have a lot of muscle. It may have nothing whatever to do with my having too much fat.

In a way you would be right. Muhammad Ali, when he was the world heavyweight boxing champion, probably weighed several stones more than the generally accepted ideal weight for his height. And yet his body probably contained no more fat than it needed. His weight was largely due to muscle bulk, and so we would not really have considered him to be overweight. But being overweight is not quite as simple as this.

First, although it is true that a boxer in peak physical condition may have no excess fat, once his training schedule is slackened a lot of that muscle tissue is quickly replaced by fat. Second (and of much greater relevance to most of us), there is no accurate or convenient way of measuring how much of our weight is made up of fat and how much of other tissues such as bone and muscle. You can get an *approximate* idea of the proportion of fat present by a simple 'pinch' test. To do this, you merely pinch a fold of skin at the back of your upper arm (behind the triceps muscle) or around your waist. This fold of skin contains a layer of fat called sub-cutaneous fat. If the fold measures an inch or more in thickness then you have too much fat. This test (which is occasionally used by doctors, sometimes using rather sophisticated calipers) serves as only a very rough guide and is generally considered to be less reliable than one of the oldest tests of all – weighing yourself.

The problem about using weight as an indication of whether or not you are overweight is that you are weighing your whole body and not just your fat (and remember that it is excess of fat that makes you overweight). But in the absence of a more reliable – or more convenient – test, measuring your weight is the most reliable way of finding out if you are overweight. In fact the method is sufficiently reliable for life assurance companies to be guided by its results. For very obvious reasons such companies are shrewd assessors of health risks and they have found that there is a close link between what a person weighs and his chances of getting – and possibly dying from – a disease that results from being overweight. The number of such diseases is pretty frightening and is the subject of Chapter 3.

People sometimes ask what the difference is between overweight, fat and obese. The answer is really quite simple. Since overweight is due to the presence of too much fat, 'overweight' and 'fat' mean the same. The word 'obese' is perhaps not quite so straightforward. It is derived from the Latin word *obesus*, which means 'that has eaten itself fat', and according to the *Oxford English Dictionary* means very fat or fleshy, or corpulent. Some authorities therefore consider the distinction between overweight and obese simply a matter of degree. They say that if you are ten per cent or more above your ideal weight you are overweight, and if you are twenty per cent above your ideal weight you are obese. But most authorities feel that this is simply playing with words. Overweight, fat and obese all mean the same.

A question that is often asked, and one that is very pertinent, is: what is meant by the 'ideal weight'? Surprising as it may seem, this is a difficult question to answer. The reason is that there is no scientific way of deciding what any one person's ideal weight should be. In any event, the concept of ideal weight begs the question, ideal for what? An ideal weight must be ideal for something. That something is health. Once again, we come back to the life assurance companies. They have assessed the number of people suffering from diseases – this being known as the incidence of those diseases – and how this corresponds with different weights. In so doing they have determined the weights which are associated with the lowest incidence of disease. And it is these weights which insurance companies (and most doctors) consider to be the ideal weights. Anyone who weighs *more* than their ideal weight has a statistically increased risk of illness or early death. But the converse is not true. In other words, someone who wants to weigh *less* than their ideal weight (perhaps because they look more attractive at that weight) will not *reduce* their health risk, because this risk has already reached its minimum at the ideal weight.

Because some people live very healthily at less than their ideal weight, for practical purposes it is more useful to use tables showing *maximum desirable weights* rather than ideal weights. (This of course assumes that you are not of low weight because of illness – a possibility that suggests itself if you find yourself losing weight without consciously eating less, and is a situation which requires a consultation with your doctor.)

One question often asked is, what is the maximum desirable weight for my age? And here lies one of the biggest fallacies to do with weight. It is a popular misconception that weight should automatically increase with age. Nothing could be more wrong. Certainly the *average* weight increases with age. This is because so many people become overweight as they grow older. But the maximum desirable weight remains constant. In other words, you should weigh the same when you are forty and when you are sixty years old as you did when you were twenty – assuming of course that at twenty you were at your maximum desirable weight. That is why, on page 174, you will find a table of maximum desirable weights, and on that page there is no mention of age other than the words 'irrespective of age'.

Being overweight is an epidemic in civilized and affluent societies and the causes of it are discussed in Chapter 2. Many doctors find that more than half the adults whom they see in their consulting rooms are overweight. Of these, only one in a hundred comes to see them because of a weight problem. The rest come for advice or treatment in connection with some other condition, although about ten per cent of those conditions are caused or aggravated by the patients being overweight. Examples of problems related to excess weight are arthritis and raised blood pressure, and these – together with the other conditions – are discussed in Chapter 3. Being overweight is not confined to adults. Today a disturbing number of children are overweight and their particular problems are discussed in Chapter 10.

Numerous studies in affluent countries have shown that more than a quarter of people in their twenties are overweight, nearly half of those in their thirties are overweight, and almost two-thirds of people over the age of forty are heavier than they should be.

Below the age of forty-five weight seems to be less of a problem with women than with men, but over this age more women than men are overweight. Many different reasons have been put forward for this sex difference, but this difference is unimportant. Much more important is the alarming number of people – irrespective of their sex – who are overweight. Alarming because the consequences can be so serious and even tragic. And since *you* are reading this book, doubtless *you* are one of those people. But, by the same token, your reading this book means that you are aware of your condition. And, what is more, you want to do something about it.

Fortunately, losing weight is easy. By the time you have finished reading this book you will realize just how easy it really is.

2

Why am I overweight?

Why am I overweight? It is surprising how often this question is asked. The answer would appear to be very simple. Being overweight results from eating too much. Yet there are many people who do not believe this. They have to be reminded that there were no fat inmates in the German concentration camps in the Second World War because there was very little food available. The question is therefore naive. Or is it?

To start with, what do we mean by eating too much? Most of us associate overeating with gluttony. We have a picture of a fat person eating his or her way through a mountain of food while the lean person hardly seems to eat enough to keep even a bird alive. Does this picture reflect the true state of affairs? Surprisingly, the answer very often is no. Comparing their appetite to that of a bird's seems to be a characteristic of fat people rather than of thin ones. Though clearly an exaggeration, the statement is not quite so absurd as it may sound. Studies have shown that many, though by no means all, overweight people actually eat less than average-sized people. And this is true even when comparing people of similar ages and with similar life styles, their type of work, sporting activities, and so on. It is especially true of children. Probably the majority of fat children eat less food than average-sized children.

However, it is important to dispel any delusions that overeating is not the cause of overweight. Although a fat person may eat less than a thin one he or she is still overeating. To understand this fact try to imagine what may be thought of as an energy equation:

energy surplus = energy input *minus* energy output

Energy input is the calories in the food we eat. Energy output is the calories our bodies burn up. The energy (or calorie) surplus is retained in our bodies as fat and is therefore weight gained. From the equation you can see that weight gain depends not only on how much food we eat but on how efficiently our bodies burn up energy. This therefore means that overweight results from a low energy output. The problem is, as will be explained later, that it is difficult for overweight people to increase their energy output by very much. Their energy output tends to remain fairly constant no matter how much they eat. Even exercise has only a small and relatively insignificant effect on energy output in obese people. So that no matter how little an overweight person eats, unless their weight is falling they are eating more than their body needs – or, to be pedantic, more than their body can burn up. And that is exactly what overeating is – eating more than your body needs.

As has been shown, what actually constitutes overeating varies from person to person depending on how efficient their bodies are at increasing energy output. Why is there such a variation?

There are many reasons. If you observe overweight people for a time, you will probably notice something significant about them: they move slowly. They move slowly when they sit down, when they stand up or when they walk about. They are less active than average-sized people. They are using less energy. But why do they move slowly? Possibly because they are overweight: a sort of vicious circle – being overweight leads to a decrease in activity which leads to an increase in weight. But it is more likely that their relative inactivity is an inherited tendency. As is described in Chapter 10, studies have shown that inherited traits probably play an important part in whether or not we are likely to become overweight.

Probably the most significant inherited problem is that of reduced metabolism. Metabolism is the sum total of all the chemical processes that occur in the body. These processes use up energy. Even in a state of complete rest and starvation, metabolism is taking place and calories are being used. If no movement (other than breathing or digestion) is taking place the amount of energy being used is known as the basal metabolic rate, or BMR for short.

This can actually be measured from determining the oxygen consumption after a twelve-hour period of complete rest and starvation. For a long time it was thought that overweight people had a low BMR compared with average-sized people. Experiments have shown that this is not usually so. The basal metabolism of most obese people is the same as that of average-sized people. It appears that the mechanism which controls the metabolic responses is defective. As an example let us look for a moment at the body's response to a meal. The intake of oxygen (which is necessary for the burning up of calories) into the blood stream through the lungs is increased and heat is produced. Thus if more food is eaten than the body needs, oxygen consumption and heat production are increased. In a person of average weight this fine control over metabolism – for convenience I shall call it the 'metabolistat' – works so well that doubling food intake may lead to only a very small increase in weight. In some overweight people it appears that this metabolistat is defective so that heat production fails to match energy input. Although this may well be an inherited defect, it is likely that obesity in infancy or childhood may also harm the metabolistat. In other words it is difficult to determine how much is cause and how much is effect.

Obesity in infancy may be the cause of reduced energy output in adulthood. This is probably the result of an increase in the number of fat cells during the first six months of life. The probable nature of this mechanism is described in Chapter 10. The point that concerns us here is that if the theory is correct that the number of fat cells is increased by infant obesity, then an adult has difficulty in burning up excess energy rather than having this deposited in the body as fat.

This tendency to convert energy into fat also seems to occur when, instead of say three moderate meals each day, a person eats one huge meal – in other words, 'gorging'. It is not clear why this happens. One possibility is that eating itself causes heat production and therefore increases energy output. The more meals that are eaten (providing that the total daily consumption of food remains the same) the greater the energy output. Another possibility is that the body simply cannot burn up the large number of calories in one huge meal and so many of these are converted into fat. Starving yourself during the day and eating one good meal in the evening is therefore a bad way to try to lose weight.

A common cause of decreased energy output is of course lack of exercise. People who leave school (where they have usually regularly taken part in active games) often become overweight unless they continue to be physically active. But the most common manifestation of decreased activity leading to obesity is the well-recognized condition of 'middle-age spread'. This occurs in many people as they grow older because, little by little, they slow down physically. At the same time their eating habits remain unchanged. Just one potato or one slice of bread more than the body needs each day can add a few ounces of weight each week. This amounts to perhaps an extra stone in weight each year. Of course exercise plays only a small role in the treatment of obesity. This is because the amount of exercise that has to be taken is enormous if a significant number of calories are to be burned up (see Chapter 8). Exercise and physical activity seem to play a more significant role in the prevention of obesity and are less important once overweight is established.

These are therefore the main ways in which energy output is decreased. The important point to remember is that no matter how low the energy output is, if the energy input exceeds it – and it may take only a very small amount of food to achieve this – your body will retain surplus energy which will be converted to fat and your weight will increase.

But of course not all overweight people have low energy outputs. Many of them have high energy inputs, while their metabolism remains normal. These are the overweight people who generally *do* eat more than normal. *Why* do they eat more? There are many reasons.

One of the most common reasons is a defective appetite-controlling mechanism. It is thought that this mechanism, often known as the 'appestat', has its centre in a part of the brain called the hypothalamus. It is sensitive to two separate sensations – hunger and satiety. The hunger part of the appetite centre is probably stimulated by low blood sugar levels (as occurs two or three hours after a meal). The rise in blood sugar after a meal depresses the activity of the satiety centre. The appetite centre is probably sensitive to other factors. A fall in body temperature, for example, stimulates it. This is probably why in cold weather we tend to eat more so that we consume more calories that can be burnt in order to keep us warm.

With such a superbly designed mechanism why is it that so many of us still manage to eat too much? What makes the appestat go wrong? The things that make it go wrong happen mainly in childhood and are discussed in Chapter 10. Briefly, the appetite centre can be overridden by higher brain centres. If this happens over a period of time the centre may become 'conditioned' in such a way that it is set at a higher level so that it takes more food than normal to depress its activity. This is particularly liable to happen if solids, especially cereals (which contain a lot of carbohydrate), are introduced too early into a baby's diet. It is also thought by some authorities that bottle-fed babies are more likely to develop defective appestats than those that are breast-fed. Also the inclusion of sugar and sweet-tasting foods in a baby's diet are likely to encourage the development of a 'sweet tooth' which in its turn leads to a high calorie consumption. Unfortunately, how babies are fed is not always entirely to blame. It is likely that some overweight people actually inherit a defective appestat, a sweet tooth or even a feature of having fewer food dislikes. These inherited traits predispose to childhood overeating. In turn, childhood overeating, whether it be due to environmental factors or inherited traits or both, may further damage the appestat. Children who overeat become fat. Fat children tend to become fat adults.

Childhood is of course not the only time that overeating happens. There are many reasons why adults eat too much even if they ate quite normally as children.

Some people eat too much because they have a psychological or psychiatric disorder. Many people who are emotionally disturbed or depressed overeat, probably because they find food comforting. Some people increase their food consumption when they are under stress rather as other people tend to bite their nails. Some people eat food all day long out of sheer boredom.

Eating food can become a habit or even an addiction. The outstanding example of this today is that when many people give up smoking they often feel a definite need to replace the habit or addiction of smoking by another – and this is usually eating. A large number of people blame their weight gain on giving up smoking. In fact, of course, their weight gain has been due to eating more and not to the lack of tobacco, but the reason for overeating is the transference of their emotional dependence from nicotine to food. Although there is probably no physical link between tobacco and weight, some authorities have claimed that after stopping smoking the bowel tends to absorb food more efficiently and therefore weight is gained.

Although obesity is a disease of affluent societies it is a curious anachronism that it is more common in the lower socio-economic groups. How much of this is due to lower educational standards and how much to the fact that fattening foods tend to be cheaper than less fattening foods is not clear but undoubtedly both are important factors.

Culture, in terms of both aestheticism and national habit, plays an important part. In most civilized countries today slimness is fashionable. In certain countries though – Italy, for example – it is considered 'fashionable', especially in the lower socio-economic groups, for a mother of a family to be plump. A striking example of this is described in *The White Nile* by Alan Moorehead. In it he describes the wives of an African chieftain who spent most of their lives sitting around a stew-pot filled with food of high calorific value. Their main activity was to constantly eat from this pot so that they would become as fat as possible – so fat that many of them could not even stand up. In Western civilization one has only to look at the paintings of Rubens and Renoir to realize that obesity was considered aesthetically attractive by many people.

Another stimulus to overeating is something which in the United States is called 'externality'. This is the tendency of some people to eat whenever they see a visual or aural stimulus, such as an advertisement or television commercial for a bar of chocolate.

There are many answers, therefore, to the question, Why am I overweight? Some answers have to do with not burning up enough calories. Others are concerned with simple gluttony, if only we were prepared to admit it to ourselves. There are inherited traits and there are environmental factors which may be important. Of course not all the reasons mentioned apply to every overweight person – far from it. But whatever the reason (or reasons) the basic cause of overweight is always the same – eating too much.

3

Does being overweight matter?

Few people today would deny the obvious advantages of a lean figure. For aesthetic reasons thinness is now fashionable, almost as if slimness were next to godliness. But, more important, people who are lean generally have more efficient bodies in terms of circulation of the blood, heart action, reflexes, co-ordination, and so on. Their physical activity and sudden bursts of energy are much better tolerated. Their potential for work and leisure activities is much greater than if they were overweight. In short, their life is likely to be more enjoyable.

Of course there is much more to slimness than this. To consider the question 'Does being overweight matter?', we have to examine the positive disadvantages of being overweight. There can be few people today who refuse to accept that obesity is a health hazard. Almost everyone knows that the answer to the question is undeniably yes. Most people know, too, some of the diseases that may be associated with obesity. But many people are amazed at the sheer number of such illnesses. Moreover, such people are often shocked to learn that obesity can cause them to die considerably earlier than they might otherwise have done.

An understanding of the extent and nature of these illnesses, together with a knowledge of the increased risk of dying young, provides a powerful motivating force for those who are wondering whether losing weight is really worth the effort. But first, a qualifying remark is needed. The conditions that will be discussed are ones that have an increased prevalence, or lead to an increased risk of dying because of a particular illness or habit among overweight people. There is therefore an *association* between obesity and these conditions. This does not necessarily mean that obesity is a direct *cause* of them. It may be that obesity simply acts as a 'catalyst' for some other factor or group of factors which is the main cause of a given condition. Alternatively obesity may simply aggravate an existing condition which would otherwise have continued to be present in a milder form. It is important to appreciate the distinction between a causal relationship and one of association. Obesity is so common and many of its associated conditions have so many different factors that may be involved in their causation that it is difficult to determine precisely the role of obesity. Obesity as a causal factor is a matter of considerable controversy in the medical profession today. And nowhere is this more true than in the first – and probably most important – diseases that will be discussed: those of the heart and blood vessels, or cardiovascular disease.

Cardiovascular disease is an umbrella term that embraces a number of diseases which are characterized by unhealthy arteries. If the arteries supplying blood to the heart are affected the condition is called coronary artery disease. If the arteries to the brain are unhealthy the condition is called cerebrovascular disease. The condition of generalized diseased arteries is known as peripheral vascular disease. A fourth variant is the condition of raised blood pressure which is called hypertension. Of course, although a person may have any one of these diseases, they are quite likely to have two, three or all four present.

In what way do the arteries become unhealthy? And why is cardiovascular disease important? Well, the inner surfaces have deposited on them lumpy deposits, consisting mainly of fatty substances. These are called atheromatous plaques and the theories of how they are formed are discussed in Chapter 6. Plaque formation leads to narrowing of the arteries with restriction of the blood flow to the tissues or organs supplied by the blood vessels. In cerebrovascular disease, where the brain is affected, this is characterized clinically by mental impairment, confusion, loss of memory, giddiness and fainting spells. If an artery becomes blocked, part of the brain is destroyed and a 'stroke' or paralysis results. In peripheral vascular disease the consequences depend upon the part of the body affected. This may be the kidneys, for example, with resultant impairment of kidney function, or the calf muscles of the leg causing pain on walking. The two most serious aspects of cardiovascular disease, however, are hypertension and coronary heart disease. Hypertension is serious because it is itself a major factor in the causation of all other types of cardiovascular disease. Coronary heart disease is serious because it is a major cause of death.

Let us look for a moment at coronary heart disease in some detail. First, what are its manifestations? If the arteries are narrowed, insufficient blood reaches the heart muscle during exertion causing a well-recognized kind of chest pain which is called 'angina pectoris'. If an artery becomes blocked a portion of heart muscle is destroyed. The blocking of the artery is called coronary thrombosis – a 'heart attack' or 'coronary' – while the destruction of heart muscle is known medically as a myocardial infarction. If such infarction is sufficiently severe to stop the heart beating, sudden death results. So coronary heart disease is manifest in one of three ways – angina, a 'coronary', or sudden death. The staggering fact is that this disease is the cause of a third of all male deaths between the ages of thirty-five and sixty-four occurring in Britain and the United States. Coronary heart disease accounts for more than half of all middle-aged deaths – deaths of men and women between the ages of forty-five and fifty-four. Compare this with cancer, which accounts for a quarter of all middle-aged deaths, or accidents, poisoning and violence, which cause much less than a tenth of deaths in this age group. You can now appreciate the importance of this disease. We do not know, however, how much obesity has to do with this. Its association is undeniable because an increase in weight by more than a fifth of his or her desirable weight increases a person's risk of dying from coronary heart disease by more than a third. Yet there is no evidence that obesity by itself causes such disease. However, it does seem to increase the risk when other risk factors are present – these other factors include hypertension, diabetes, physical inactivity and a high level of fats (cholesterol and triglycerides especially) in the blood. Of course, obesity is itself associated with an increased prevalence of each of these factors. It is clear, therefore, that there are many factors which are closely interwoven, and one of these is obesity.

The risk of dying because of a disease – or the mortality from a disease – has been determined by life assurance companies. Detailed actuarial statistics give indisputable evidence that obesity increases the likelihood of an early death. For example, the increased mortality from cardiovascular and kidney disease is about fifty per cent. Diabetes of middle age – 'maturity onset' diabetes – has been found to have a fourfold increase in mortality in overweight people. Of course it is not only the mortality but also the prevalence of many diseases that is increased with obesity. Maturity onset diabetes is an example of a disease with not only an increased mortality but an increased prevalence in overweight people. Another is cirrhosis of the liver. This disease, which has a mortality two and a half that of the average, may be more common in obesity because many sufferers are alcoholics: and as alcohol contains a lot of calories, consumption of a large quantity of it predisposes to obesity.

Gallstones seem to be more common in overweight people. This may be something to do with high cholesterol levels (which are more prevalent in obese people) as many gallstones are made largely of cholesterol. The classic observation that all doctors remember as medical students is that a typical patient with gall-bladder disease or gallstones is female, forty, fertile, fecund – and fat! Another surgical condition, appendicitis, is claimed by some authorities to be more common in overweight people. There appears to be little evidence for this, but it is certain that the mortality from both appendicitis and gallstones is, for each, about two and a half that of the average. The increased mortality probably has less to do with the basic condition, but more to do with the complications of operating on an obese patient and problems that can arise in the post-operative period. There are clear reasons why operations can be hazardous for an overweight person. There is the obvious technical difficulty for the surgeon who, particularly in an abdominal operation, has to 'wade through' layers of greasy fat before reaching the diseased organ. Once inside the abdominal cavity dissection may be hampered by the presence of fat. Respiration may present anaesthetic problems because the diaphragm in an obese patient works less efficiently in the movements for breathing because it is heavily infiltrated with fat. Not only does this increase the risk of death during the operation but there is a greater likelihood of post-operative chest infection. The period immediately following surgery is further complicated by an increased prevalence in the obese patient of thrombosis of the deep-lying veins of the calves. This may result in a clot being 'thrown off' and passed along the veins to the blood vessels of the lungs, such a clot being known as a pulmonary embolus. This can cause destruction of lung tissue which, if sufficiently large, may be fatal.

Deep vein thrombosis is more likely to occur in overweight people because varicose veins (a condition which increases the likelihood of thrombosis) is more common in obesity. So, too, is inflammation and minor clot formation, known as thrombophlebitis or, more popularly, 'phlebitis'. This brings me to the large number of conditions which, though they do not account for an increased mortality, are more common and cause more suffering in those who are overweight. Perhaps the most obvious is arthritis. This is a term used to describe inflammation of joints, and there are numerous causes such as rheumatoid arthritis, infection and gout. What I am particularly referring to, however, is simple 'wear and tear' of the weight-bearing joints – the spine, the hips and the knees. It is not difficult to see that extra weight is likely to speed up the normal 'wearing out' process with resultant stiffness and pain. For the same reason overweight children are more likely to have knock-knees and flat feet. In addition, fractures and severe limb injuries seem to occur more often in obese people. This is possibly at least in part the result of the extra weight they are carrying. An additional factor, however, is that overweight people are more accident-prone and clumsy. This seems to apply especially to fat women who have an increased mortality (compared with normal weight women) from accidents of about fifty per cent.

Women who are overweight are more prone to a number of conditions. The most common are probably complications of pregnancy and labour. These include toxaemia of pregnancy, a condition usually manifested by raised blood pressure and fluid retention and a risk of epileptic fits. The complications of labour result in an increase in perinatal mortality. Another result of obesity is interference with the normal functioning of the ovaries. This leads to infrequent or non-existent ovulation – the release from the ovaries of eggs. This causes the absence of menstrual periods but, more important, lack of ovulation makes a woman unable to conceive and therefore infertile. In older women, obesity is associated with an increased prevalence of womb prolapse (the supporting muscles of the pelvic floor being very lax) and cancer of the body (as distinct from the cervix or neck) of the womb.

Obesity is associated with an increased tendency, in both men and women, of a number of conditions of the abdomen and the digestive tract. Because the muscles tend to be lax and infiltrated by fatty tissue, hernias (or ruptures) are more common. These may be in the groin or around the navel. They may also arise from the site of a surgical incision. There is also an internal hernia in which the top end of the stomach slides into the chest from the abdomen through a weakness (caused by fatty infiltration) in the muscles of the diaphragm. This condition, known as hiatus hernia (and which incidentally is far more common in women than in men), usually causes regurgitation of stomach acid into the gullet and may be very painful. Overweight people seem to be prone to having piles, diverticulitis (see Chapter 5) and cancer of the large bowel.

It was mentioned earlier in this chapter that obese people are more likely to have post-operative chest infections. But quite apart from surgery those who are overweight are more prone to coughs and bronchial conditions, and unfortunately this applies equally to children. Also obesity is associated with an increased tendency to breathlessness on exertion. This is probably due to a combination of weak muscles of the diaphragm and rib cage because of fatty infiltration and the greater strain on the heart.

Of course there are many other conditions associated with obesity, such as various kinds of inflammation of the skin, skin infections (boils, for example) and hirsutism (an increase in un-wanted bodily hair). You may find it surprising therefore to know that there are some conditions which are actually *less* common among obese people. There are two in particular – peptic ulcers and suicide. Why is this? It may be because obese people suffer less stress, or have a more cheerful disposition, than many other people. And stress is a definite factor in the causation of peptic ulcers, particularly duodenal ulcers. Clearly stress is a fundamental factor in most suicides.

Having said that many fat people have a cheerful disposition, one must not be blind to the fact that obesity, and many of the conditions associated with obesity, are the cause of considerable physical discomfort and therefore general misery and unhappiness and a loss of working time. There can be little doubt that being overweight matters – and it matters very much.

4

All about calories

You are unlikely to open any slimming book or magazine without finding the word 'calories' mentioned constantly. This is not at all surprising since all methods of losing weight by dietary means are concerned with reducing our intake of calories.

A calorie, quite simply, is a unit of energy. Energy is the capacity to do work, and it may take the form of heat, light, electricity and so on. It can never be destroyed but merely converted from one form to another. An obvious example is the mechanical energy of a waterfall (or hydraulic dam) being converted into electricity which in its turn may be changed into heat or light.

Our bodies need energy and food is the fuel that provides the source of this energy. In round figures one gram of carbohydrate provides four calories, one gram of fat nine calories, one gram of protein four calories, and one gram of alcohol yields seven calories. There are various ways in which the calorific content of food can be measured. One method consists of placing a sample of weighed food in a 'bomb' which is filled with pure oxygen. The bomb is then placed in an outer container which has a measured amount of water in it. The food in the bomb is then burned, the heat produced causing a rise in temperature of the water in the container. The calorific value of the food that has been burned can be calculated from the result. One calorie is the heat required to raise the temperature of one kilogram (approximately 2·2 pints) of water one degree centigrade. Strictly speaking this is a kilocalorie but for simplicity it is conventionally referred to as a calorie. (Scientists and nutritionists now use a different unit of energy called a joule, one calorie being equivalent to 4·2 joules. However, in non-technical publications the calorie is the unit that is likely to be used for a long time to come.)

Of course food is not pure carbohydrate, pure fat or pure protein. It is a combination of two or all three nutrients. For example, 25 grams of white bread (just under one ounce) contains about 14 grams of carbohydrate, one gram of fat and two grams of protein. Its total calorific value can be worked out thus:

Carbohydrate	14 x 4 =	56 calories
Fat	1 x 9 =	9 calories
Protein	2 x 4 =	8 calories
Total		73 calories

But a more detailed discussion of the calorific value of common foods will be left to Chapter 17.

Our bodies need energy for many reasons. In the first place we need energy simply to live. By this is meant the involuntary movements, such as heartbeat and breathing, which go on all the time every minute of each day. A lot of energy is also needed to maintain the body temperature. The energy used in these essential processes is called basal metabolism. An average man needs about 1500 calories a day for his basal metabolism. An average woman (who weighs less) needs about 1300 calories a day. It is perhaps difficult to visualize these amounts of energy. An easy way is to realize that the same energy would boil sufficient water to provide about 200 cups of tea each day!

But we need energy not only for basal metabolism but also for all the voluntary activities that we do each day – standing, dressing, washing, walking, and so on. The number of calories we need depends on the kind of activity. Light work of a domestic nature uses up three calories each minute: a similar rate of expenditure occurs in a game of golf. Moderately heavy work (such as gardening) or a not too vigorous game of tennis (or, if you prefer, disco dancing) burns up six calories a minute. Heavy work (such as coal-mining) or football or competitive swimming uses up ten or more calories a minute.

Table: Recommended Daily Intakes of Energy
for the UK *(Department of Health and Social Security, 1969)*

Age range[a]	Occupational category	Body weight[c] kg	lb*	Energy[d] kcals†	mJ[e]
BOYS AND GIRLS					
0 up to 1 year[b]		7·3	16	800	3·3
1 up to 2 years		11·4	25	1200	5·0
2 up to 3 years		13·5	30	1400	5·9
3 up to 5 years		16·5	36	1600	6·7
5 up to 7 years		20·5	45	1800	7·5
7 up to 9 years		25·1	55	2100	8·8
BOYS					
9 up to 12 years		31·9	70	2500	10·5
12 up to 15 years		45·5	100	2800	11·7
15 up to 18 years		61·0	134	3000	12·6
GIRLS					
9 up to 12 years		33·0	73	2300	9·6
12 up to 15 years		48·6	107	2300	9·6
15 up to 18 years		56·1	123	2300	9·6
MEN					
18 up to 35 years	Sedentary	65	143	2700	11·3
	Moderately active	65	143	3000	12·6
	Very active	65	143	3600	15·1
35 up to 65 years	Sedentary	65	143	2600	10·9
	Moderately active	65	143	2900	12·1
	Very active	65	143	3600	15·1
65 up to 75 years }	Assuming a	63	139	2350	9·8
75 and over	sedentary life	63	139	2100	8·8
WOMEN					
18 up to 55 years	Most occupations	55	121	2200	9·2
	Very active	55	121	2500	10·5
55 up to 75 years }	Assuming a	53	117	2050	8·6
75 and over	sedentary life	53	117	1900	8·0
Pregnancy (4th month onwards)				2400	10·0
Breast-feeding				2700	11·3

The calorie expenditure by an average man has been worked out by nutritionists for almost every conceivable activity. There are various ways that calorie expenditure can be measured and the most usual involves determining the volume of oxygen used during activity – energy being produced as a result of the oxidation of foodstuffs. The calories that have been burned up can be calculated from the volume of oxygen consumed. The energy requirements for every occupation are known and so the total number of calories needed each day can be worked out. Let us see for a moment how this is done.

An average man spends eight hours in bed – just over 60 calories an hour. He spends a further eight hours in non-occupational pursuits – these can vary from 100 to 225 but on average are a little over 160 calories an hour. The final eight hours he spends at work. If this is sedentary (office worker, teacher, lawyer, doctor, for example) he will burn up about 100 calories per hour. If he is moderately active (postman, bus conductor, plumber, light industrial worker) he will use 150 calories an hour. And if he is very active (coal-miner, forestry worker) he will use 225

---

[a] The ages are from one birthday to another: e.g. 9 up to 12 is from the ninth up to, but not including, the twelfth birthday. The figures in the Table in general refer to the mid-point of the ranges, though those for the range 18 up to 35 refer to the age 25 years, and for the range 18 up to 55, to 35 years of age.

[b] Average figures relating to the first year of life.

[c] The body weights of children and adolescents are averages and relate to London in 1965. (Taken from Tanner, Whitehouse and Takashi, 1966; Tables IVA and IVB, 50th centile.)

[d] Average requirements relating to groups of individuals.

[e] Megajoules (10 joules). Calculated from the relation 1 kilocalorie = 4·186 kilojoules, and rounded to 1 decimal place.

* Official lbs units are not published by the DHSS. The figures given are the author's own conversions.

† A *kilocalorie* is the correct name for what, in general use, is often referred to as a *calorie*.

calories each hour. So the total energy expenditure for the 24-hour period is:

	Sedentary	Moderately active	Very active
8 hours in bed	500	500	500
8 hours non-occupation	1300	1300	1300
8 hours working	900	1200	1800
24 hours total calories	2700	3000	3600

Of course these round figures are only average ones since energy requirements depend upon very many factors. Heavy people need more energy than smaller people, although the difference is not directly related to body size since heavy people are often less active than slimmer ones. People who are more active also need more energy which is one reason why children (who generally are very active) need a lot of energy. Another reason that energy requirements in childhood are high is that this is an important period of growth. Another growth period is pregnancy, and the succeeding breast-feeding makes enormous demands on energy requirements – about an extra 1000 calories a day.

There are also individual variations, regardless of the factors I have just described, in the efficiency with which each of us burns up calories (see Chapters 3 and 10). Then there are a number of hormone diseases which may affect calorie expenditure. An overactive thyroid gland, for example, causes an increase in energy output whereas an underactive thyroid decreases energy output.

Finally, the temperature of our surroundings is an important factor. In hot weather, when the body has to work less hard to keep warm, we burn up fewer calories than when the weather is cold.

For interest's sake this chapter contains a table showing the daily intakes of energy as recommended by the Department of Health and Social Security in 1969. These, of course, assume average energy requirements and it must be remembered that individual requirements may vary widely.

Do not try to remember the figures in the above table. What is much more important to remember is that if you are overweight (which most of you reading this book will be) you are eating more calories than your body needs.

5

Fibre – a food fad?

John Buchan once said that all that was needed to write a good story was to think of three totally unrelated people or things and find a way of linking them together. Consider then tooth decay, heart disease and bowel cancer. Three unrelated conditions, and serious ones at that. Ask most people to find a link between them and they would probably laugh at you. But a link there may well be and the story of its discovery is one of the most fascinating in twentieth-century medicine.

During the Second World War a British surgeon captain found that by giving bran to the men aboard his battleship he was able to relieve and prevent the constipation that was so common. He was not the first person to have noticed a link between bran and bowel action. Such an association had been noted by a number of people for many years prior to this but, perhaps because the bowel is not the most glamorous of subjects, very little had been written about it. The naval officer was, however, the first person to make any impact with his discovery. It took two distinguished British surgeons, working independently, to bring it to the notice of the world in the 1960s. One, Denis Burkitt, who had already made an international name for himself with the discovery of a quite unrelated malignant condition in Africa, noticed that Africans who had been eating the same kind of diet for centuries rarely developed a number of diseases which included tooth decay, heart disease and bowel cancer. This contrasted markedly with those Africans who were living in more urban communities and eating more Western refined diets, for these people seemed much more prone to develop those particular diseases. The other surgeon, Neil S. Painter, using

37

medical investigation techniques, mainly X-rays with radio-opaque materials, demonstrated the action on the bowel of the substance that provides the link.

So what is this substance? Mention has already been made of bran and fibre. But how can this possibly provide the link between unrelated diseases? It hardly gains credulity when you consider precisely what it is. Take wheat, for example. If this is stored for any length of time it becomes bad. The reason for this is quite simple. A wheat seed is composed of endosperm (the starch) which gives flour. It also has a small amount of germ (consisting mainly of fat and protein) and an outer wall (the husk or bran). Stored wheat becomes bad because the fat in the germ turns rancid. To stop this happening wheat has to be ground, or milled, to remove the wheatgerm. This process – refining – also removes the fibrous outer wall, the bran.

But is bran important enough to provide the link? Further examination of it would seem unlikely to persuade you otherwise. Bran, which forms the wall not just of wheat but of all plant cells, is made of indigestible carbohydrates. This means that it enters and leaves the digestive tract completely intact. Unless a substance is absorbed from the alimentary tract it cannot really be considered to have entered the body. So here is a substance – bran or fibre – which never actually enters our bodies and is therefore of abso-lutely no nutritional value. And one is asked to believe that it is so important?

But fibre, or rather the lack of it, is very significant. Fibre deficiency is perhaps the most common deficiency condition in the world – certainly in the civilized and affluent world. What, however, has all this to do with slimming? Well, of course, the three diseases mentioned at the beginning of this chapter are only some of the conditions that are thought to be linked to fibre deficiency. Others include peptic ulcers, gallstones, diverticulitis, hiatus hernia, varicose veins, appendicitis and piles – and obesity.

To understand how a non-nutrient which is not even absorbed into our bodies can be so important it is useful to consider two things. First, what happens to fibre when it is inside the alimentary canal and, second, what happens to our diet when fibre is lacking.

In the alimentary tract plant fibres absorb water so that they swell and become bulky. Also they probably interfere with the absorption of certain other dietary constituents, in particular, cholesterol. Lack of fibre means that we are eating a refined diet, the part that is refined being the starches and the sugars. The theory is that because they are refined, the carbohydrates are more concentrated and more of them are eaten than in an unrefined diet.

It must be emphasized that at present a direct causal relationship between lack of dietary fibre and the diseases and conditions that will be described has not yet been proved. As with dietary fats and coronary heart disease (see Chapter 6) the link is one purely of association. Most of the evidence is based on observation of populations who have different eating habits particularly with regard to the presence or absence of fibre. There are of course many other factors which may differ in these populations, such as stress, exercise, smoking and other dietary factors. But the circumstantial evidence, particularly with regard to bowel conditions, is sufficiently strong for the fibre content to be taken seriously.

Taken in chronological order, the first parts of the alimentary tract that may be affected by the presence or absence of dietary fibre are our teeth and gums. It is thought that dental caries (tooth decay) and gum disease may be caused or aggravated by a refined diet. Saliva produces a microscopic layer of protein on tooth enamel. Sugar encourages the growth of bacteria which converts this protein layer into a thick, slimy substance called plaque. Refined flour makes this plaque an adhesive pasty substance which retains the sugar, which in turn by the action of the bacteria produces acids which destroy the tooth enamel.

The stomach is the next part of the digestive tract which it is thought may be affected by lack of dietary fibre. The lack of bulk in the mouth causes less mastication (chewing) to take place. Since mastication stimulates saliva secretion, lack of fibre results in poor saliva production. As the saliva is swallowed and enters the stomach, a shortage of it may lead to a loss of a 'buffering' effect on the stomach acids, with resultant peptic ulceration of the stomach or duodenum – a gastric or duodenal ulcer.

The large bowel (or colon) is the next part of the alimentary tract to be directly affected by lack of dietary fibre. Here we are on much less theoretical ground as the evidence from various investigation techniques is very impressive. The crux of the matter is that lack of fibre causes the formation of small viscid faeces. It has been well demonstrated that small faeces lead to lack of motility of the bowel so that the faeces are moved along very slowly – a condition sometimes referred to as faecal arrest. In addition, the absence of adequate bulk in the bowel and poor motility causes the muscles of the bowel wall to contract vigorously in a segmental fashion so that there are pockets of greatly increased pressure within the cavity (or lumen) of the bowel. The increased pressure results in herniation, or rupture, of the mucosal lining through the surrounding muscle layers, forming pouches called diverticulae – a condition known as diverticulosis. Inevitably these pouches become infected and inflamed – a condition known as diverticulitis, characterized by abdominal pain, variable constipation or diarrhoea, and the passage of blood in the faeces. Diverticulitis may become a serious condition since it can lead to abscess formation, bowel obstruction and concern because of the difficulty in distinguishing it from bowel cancer.

The vigorous contraction of the muscles of the bowel wall may be very painful even in the absence of diverticulitis. In fact, in the absence of proven disease (generally by X-rays using contrast media, for example, barium enema X-rays) this condition, which though not serious can be a considerable nuisance that is surprisingly common, has been aptly called the 'irritable bowel syndrome'. Diverticulosis (and its subsequent diverticulitis) are diseases of middle-age which may be prevented by a high-fibre diet taken over a period of years. Irritable bowel syndrome can often be relieved by a high-fibre diet.

The faecal arrest, mentioned earlier, is thought to be important in the causation of two important diseases of the bowel – acute appendicitis and cancer of the bowel. Faecal arrest causes the formation of a small hard faecal mass, called faecolith, which obstructs the appendix and leads to its inflammation and hence appendicitis.

The role of faecal arrest in the causation of large bowel cancer is a little more complex, although at the present time it is still somewhat speculative. It is thought that Western diets lead to the formation of bowel bacteria which degrade bile salts (which are secreted into the bowel from the gallbladder via the bile duct) into carcinogenic – potentially cancer-producing – substances. Faecal arrest causes these carcinogenic substances to remain in contact with the bowel mucosa for a long time, and hence there is an increased tendency towards the formation of cancer of the large bowel.

Of course the most obvious manifestation of lack of bowel motility and faecal arrest is one of the commonest of human symptoms – constipation. And it is not difficult to see that there is a relationship between constipation and diverticulitis, appendicitis and bowel cancer – a sobering thought indeed. But apart from the effects of constipation on the bowel there are other conditions which are believed by some doctors to be attributable to constipation. Consider for a moment the immediate short-term consequence of constipation. It is, to use a medical colloquial expression, 'straining at stool' (a delightfully descriptive phrase, if lacking in finesse). This causes a rise in the intra-abdominal pressure. Such increases in abdominal pressure can be transmitted along the veins of the legs (causing varicose veins and the associated condition of deep vein thrombosis) and along the rectal veins (causing internal piles). Also, at the upper part of the abdomen, the increase in abdominal pressure can affect the anatomical relationship between the lower end of the oesophagus (or gullet) and the stomach, causing reflux of acid from the stomach up the oesophagus and a condition known as hiatus hernia.

In addition to the mechanical effects of fibre, or its lack, in the bowel, there are theories about its effects on the absorption of certain dietary constituents, in particular, cholesterol. An increase in the absorption of cholesterol from the bowel, as probably happens when dietary fibre is low, causes a rise in the blood level of cholesterol. Many gallstones are formed from cholesterol and there appears to be a link therefore between lack of dietary fibre and gallstones and gallbladder disease.

As is discussed in Chapter 6, there is a definite relationship between high blood cholesterol and coronary artery disease. There may therefore also be a link between eating refined foods and heart disease. This may result not only from the increased absorption of cholesterol from the bowel but also from the increased calorie consumption that may occur on a refined diet. The absorption of large amounts of calories from the bowel increases the manufacture of cholesterol in the liver, and this cholesterol enters the blood in addition to the dietary cholesterol.

If we wander more into the realm of theoretical fancy we see that diabetes is another disease which it is thought may have a link with lack of dietary fibre. Again, this disease supposedly results from the absorption of large quantities of sugar which happens because a refined diet leads to high concentrations of sugar in the bowel. Why this may be a factor in the causation of diabetes has not been demonstrated. The theory is that high concentrations of refined sugar are absorbed from the bowel much more rapidly than sugar in the unrefined state. These high concentrations lead to sudden and large variations in the level of blood sugar rather than a more steady level with gentle fluctuations. It is thought that the sudden high blood sugar levels, or 'peaks', in some way damage the pancreas over a period of time. The pancreas contains cells, called the Islets of Langerhans, which produce insulin, the hormone responsible for ensuring a stable blood sugar level. With progressive damage to the pancreas, insulin production becomes deficient. It is possible therefore that a refined diet is at least a contributory factor in the causation of diabetes among young people. It may also be a factor in diabetes that occurs for the first time in middle-age. But since middle or late onset diabetes usually occurs in overweight people, it is probable that there is merely a relative lack of insulin for the excess tissue present in an obese person. And this brings us to the link between fibre and overweight.

What precisely is the link? And how, is it claimed, can fibre help us to lose weight? We have already seen that a diet lacking in fibre is abundant in refined carbohydrates. Refined carbohydrates have a small volume and are not very filling, and so we eat more of them than if they were unrefined. For example, 30 grams (1 oz) of sweets is much less filling than two raw apples, and yet the carbohydrate content is similar. So, simply by providing more bulk an unrefined diet will lead to the consumption of less energy than a refined diet. Therefore, it is claimed, if you change from a refined to an unrefined diet you will lose weight.

Reducing the consumption of carbohydrates is not the only way that fibre is supposed to help in weight-reduction. By increasing the motility of the bowel less carbohydrate is absorbed. Also unrefined carbohydrates take longer to be digested in the bowel. So less carbohydrate will be broken down into sugar and this, too, will cause less carbohydrate absorption.

The increased bulk of a high-fibre diet means that we chew more. If food has to be chewed for a longer time before it can be swallowed, less of it is likely to be eaten. Also the process of chewing increases saliva production and secretion by the salivary glands. This saliva is swallowed and possibly contributes to the feeling of fullness in the stomach.

How is fibre eaten? Well, there is a lot of fibre or roughage present in nuts, fruit and leafy vegetables. The best source, however, is cereals, and many (though not all) breakfast cereals are now made from the outer layers of wheat. An increasing amount of bread made from wholemeal flour is now available, too. Pure wheat bran, in the form of bran flakes, can now be bought at many health food and chemist shops.

How much fibre should be eaten? This is a difficult question to answer because the amount of fibre needed varies from person to person and it is often impossible to measure the fibre present in food. Substituting wholemeal for refined flour bread, whole-wheat cereal for ordinary cereal and similar modifications may be all that is necessary. If you prefer – or in addition – two or more tablespoons of bran sprinkled over your breakfast cereal or mixed with milk, for example, can be taken each day.

To return to the original question, Is fibre the new food fad? Or is it simply a lot of fanciful nonsense? As is discussed in Chapter 6, the fact that no direct causal link has yet been demonstrated between dietary fat and coronary heart disease does not mean that the possibility should be thrown out of the window. Similarly the lack of *proof* of a direct link between dietary fibre and a number of diseases does not mean that the importance of fibre should be completely dismissed. Lack of scientific evidence has, however, persuaded some doctors and nutritionists to adopt what many other doctors feel to be cavalier attitudes. Just as the circumstantial evidence linking dietary fat and coronary heart disease is very strong, so a similar kind of evidence between fibre and certain diseases is sufficiently impressive for us to give it serious consideration. In particular, certain conditions and diseases of the bowel (such as constipation, piles and diverticulitis) are almost certainly helped or prevented by dietary fibre.

6

Cholesterol – just a theory?

One question that is often asked is, Should I cut down on cholesterol? This is, in fact, not one, but many questions. What the person asking it wants to know is – What is cholesterol? Do I eat cholesterol or does my body make it from certain constituents of my food? If so, what are those constituents? What effects does cholesterol have in my body? In particular, does it affect my heart?

First, let us see exactly what cholesterol is. It is a fatty substance which is present in everyone's blood. The problem is that it does not just stay in the blood itself. It can be deposited in the lining of our arteries and this leads to the narrowing of such arteries. Cholesterol is also an important constituent of lumpy deposits on the inner lining surfaces of arteries. These deposits, known as atheromatous plaques, can cause narrowing of the arteries and eventually, sometimes, blockage.

If the arteries that are affected by such narrowing or blockage supply blood to a vital organ serious damage will occur. If the arteries supplying the brain, for example, are diseased, the reduction in blood flow leads to a general impairment of mental faculties – forgetfulness, poor concentration and deterioration of memory – and possibly episodes of giddiness or fainting. If there is an actual blockage brain tissue is damaged and an affected person has what is commonly called a 'stroke'. Similarly, if the arteries supplying blood to our kidneys are affected these vital organs may be damaged, causing serious illness.

The most vital organ that may be affected by damaged arteries is the heart – the large muscular pump which drives blood around the body. Heart muscle, like any other living tissue, needs oxygen

45

which it receives via blood vessels called coronary arteries. During physical exertion, if the coronary arteries are narrowed, insufficient blood reaches the heart muscle. The resulting oxygen lack causes chest pain – angina pectoris. In extreme cases the bore of the artery becomes so small that it eventually becomes blocked. When this happens no blood (and therefore no oxygen) can reach the portion of heart muscle supplied by that artery and the muscle tissue is destroyed – coronary thrombosis. Alternatively, coronary thrombosis (or a 'heart attack') may result from a small blood clot occurring in an artery already narrowed by the deposition of fatty substances in its lining.

What causes atheromatous plaques to be formed in arteries, particularly in the coronary arteries? Many factors are believed to play a part – smoking, overweight, high blood pressure, lack of exercise and stress being among the most important. Another factor is cholesterol. The question is whether our diet has a direct effect on whether or not we get coronary heart disease. This has been the subject of considerable research for many years, and yet we still do not know all the answers.

But let us look at what we *do* know. We know that people whose diet contains a lot of saturated fatty acids and cholesterol tend to have high blood levels of cholesterol. We also know that people with high blood cholesterol levels have an increased chance of dying from coronary heart disease – the risk is about double that of a person with a normal level. We know, too, that people with coronary heart disease tend to have high blood cholesterol levels. From what has been said it may seem at first glance quite obvious that a diet high in saturated fats and cholesterol will increase your chance of dying from coronary heart disease. But this is not necessarily so.

It is known, and it has been demonstrated, that a high saturated fat diet increases the level of blood cholesterol. (It has also been shown that a high dietary cholesterol content will tend to have the same effect, but not so markedly because the body is able to synthesize a lot of cholesterol itself if cholesterol is absent in the diet.) But the link between a high blood cholesterol level and coronary heart disease is one of association only. The classic observation is that Japanese men who come to live in San Francisco acquire high blood cholesterol levels and have an increased tendency to coronary heart disease in similar proportions to those of the native population. This is in sharp contrast to the low cholesterol levels and only a small tendency to heart disease of the indigenous population of Japan. But this does not *prove* that such acquired high blood cholesterol levels have increased the risk of heart disease. There could be some other factor which is affected by a high saturated fat diet. Such a factor could have two different and unrelated consequences – the one being the high blood cholesterol levels and the other the increased risk of heart disease.

Of course it would be both handy and tidy to demonstrate a direct causal relationship between high blood cholesterol and coronary heart disease. This would complete a beautifully simple chain of events: high saturated fat diet leads to high blood cholesterol which leads to coronary heart disease. It could then be stated quite emphatically that a diet low in saturated fats would significantly reduce the risk of coronary heart disease.

Why therefore has it not been possible to demonstrate a direct link? There are three main reasons. First, it is impossible (at present, at least) to determine the extent of atheromatous disease. Of course we know the incidence of angina and coronary thrombosis because these conditions have symptoms which make them painfully apparent. But atheromatous disease is present in many people who have no symptoms. Whereas it takes only a simple blood test to determine the blood level of cholesterol – and hence the proportion of any population that has a high level – there is no test for atheromatous disease (unless you consider a post-mortem to be a test).

The second problem is that there are so many factors in the causation of coronary heart disease – smoking, high blood pressure, overweight, stress and lack of exercise being the most important. Furthermore, many of the factors are interrelated. For example, it has been shown that regular exercise can lower a previously high blood cholesterol level. There is no way of determining the relative significance of each factor, and this applies to blood cholesterol.

47

The third problem is that fats and cholesterol are not the only dietary constituents that affect blood cholesterol levels. A comparative study of Yemenite Jews living in Yemen and those living in Israel yielded interesting observations in the early 1960s. Both populations eat the same amount of saturated fats. Yet the blood cholesterol levels and the incidence of coronary heart disease were much lower in the Yemenites than in the Israelis. It was also noticed that the amount of carbohydrate eaten was the same in both groups. It emerged, however, that whereas the Yemenites ate no sucrose (simple sugar) about one-fifth of the carbohydrate eaten by the Israelis was in the form of sucrose. Another interesting observation is that the incidence of coronary heart disease in the United States has increased throughout this century together with an increase in the consumption of sucrose. The total amount of carbohydrates consumed has fallen as has the consumption of saturated fats.

If what emerges is a complex picture then you have an accurate assessment of current medical thinking. Diet and coronary heart disease are linked. There is an association between dietary saturated fats and heart disease but, as was described above, there are populations where the incidence of such disease is high and the consumption of dietary saturated fat is not high. Complex carbohydrates – such as starch (as in potatoes) – have little effect on blood cholesterol levels, whereas simple carbohydrates such as sucrose – sugar – seem to have a significant effect on both blood cholesterol and coronary heart disease.

So what conclusions should we draw? As no link between diet and heart disease has been demonstrated scientifically, can we dismiss the whole question of cholesterol? Well, the historical and geographical evidence is rather impressive and provides a compelling, if circumstantial, case for considering our diet very carefully. The American Heart Association recommends that at least half of our dietary fat (which accounts for about forty per cent of our total calorie intake) should be in the form of unsaturated fats, and that our total dietary fat should be reduced. In Britain, in 1974, the Department of Health also recommended the reduction of our intake of saturated fats. They made no recommendations about polyunsaturated fats. But in 1976 the Royal College of Physicians of London and the British Cardiac Society did go so far as to advise that, in addition to reducing our consumption of saturated fats, we should substitute at least part of them by polyunsaturated fats. In addition, many authorities have advised the reduction of sucrose consumption. This is partly because of the relationship between dietary sucrose and blood cholesterol but also of course because sucrose is very fattening, and fat people are more likely to die from heart disease than normal weight people.

Some of you may be wondering what cholesterol (and sugar) has to do with a book concerned with obesity and slimming, particularly a book that advocates eating the foods you normally eat, but just a little less of them, rather than changing your foods to fit in with a diet. In answer, it must first be made clear that there is no suggestion that you *must* follow a modified fat and low cholesterol diet since such a modified diet would be a departure from the basic principles of simply eating less of what you normally eat in order to lose weight. But for health reasons it is wise to make *some* reductions in animal fat, such as trimming the visible fat off meat and consuming less dairy products. The significant point with regard to weight control is that fat is a highly concentrated source of calories – nine calories per gram or about 260 calories per ounce. If you cut down on fat you will also be cutting down on calories. Of course a low animal fat diet does not necessarily imply a saving of calories. For example, substituting a soft polyunsaturated fat margarine for butter will mean that you eat the same number of calories. But if you spread *less* butter on your bread and leave it at that you will save calories. Incidentally, not all soft margarines are low in saturated fats – only those that actually state that they are high in polyunsaturates and contain no cholesterol.

As regards sugar, since this has no nutritional value (apart from being rich in calories), and because there is strong evidence about its health risks, it seems sensible to reduce its consumption. Many people find that if they gradually reduce the amount of sugar they use it is only a matter of time before they find that they do not miss it at all. A good start is to reduce the amount of sugar you add to tea or coffee. Try cutting down by one teaspoon – or even half a teaspoon – each week until you find yourself quite happy with no sugar at all. If you do this you will find yourself less tempted by a whole variety of sweet and fattening foods such as cakes and biscuits. If you find it impossible to cut out your desire for sweet tastes, then switch to artificial sweeteners. As well as tablets these are available in liquid and powder forms, which makes it easy to use artificial sweeteners on breakfast cereals or strawberries. They can also be used in cooking. Some people dislike their taste at first but it is surprising how quickly a taste for them can be acquired.

Below is a list of foods which are high in cholesterol or saturated fat content. You will find a few examples of calorie-saving mentioned. These are merely meant to illustrate how eating less of these foods can help you to lose weight. By referring to the calorie tables in Chapter 17 you can readily find other examples yourself.

Foods containing a lot of cholesterol:
- eggs (especially the yolks. Don't forget that eggs are used in cooking, for example, in omelettes, soufflés, cakes)
- cream (an extra bonus being that every 30 grams (1 oz) not eaten is 250 calories saved)
- offal, that is, liver, liver pâtés, kidney, brain, heart, sweetbread
- certain seafoods such as cod-liver oil, caviare, roe, shellfish, for example, crab, lobster, shrimps

Food containing a lot of saturated fats:
- fatty meats, sausages, salami, luncheon meats, corned beef, duck, goose, poultry skin, the visible fat of meat (every 30 grams (1 oz) cut off saving 260 calories)
- whole milk (pasteurized, homogenized, evaporated, condensed) and its products such as yoghurt, butter, margarine (other than those made with polyunsaturated fats), whole milk cheeses (such as cream cheese, Cheddar, Cheshire, Stilton) and whole milk drinks (such as chocolate and milk shakes). Many calories can be saved using skimmed milk (180 calories saved per pint) and low fat milk products such as low fat yoghurt (saving 45 calories per 140 gram (5 oz) portion), low fat cheese (such as cottage cheese, a

45 gram (1½ oz) portion of which saves 135 calories compared with, say, Cheddar cheese) or medium fat cheese (such as Edam)
- coconuts, peanuts, cashew nuts
- vegetables tinned in sauces (such as baked beans)
- vegetables prepared or cooked in saturated fats (such as potato salad and potato crisps)
- puddings, cakes and biscuits made with whole milk, fats or eggs (such as pancakes, suet pudding, doughnuts and most biscuits). Also ice cream (for which the substitution of sorbet can save over 100 calories in a 55 gram (2 oz) portion). Puddings made from skimmed milk (custard, blancmange, for example) or egg whites (meringues) and jellies contain much less saturated fat and fewer calories
- chocolate, toffees, fudge, caramel
- salad cream and mayonnaise (unless the mayonnaise is made from a polyunsaturated oil)

When you cook meat discard the fat and avoid greasy gravies. Avoid frying (see Chapter 14 for examples of the number of calories saved), but if you do fry, avoid using margarine, lard, dripping, cooking fat, butter, olive and coconut oil. Either fry the food in its own fat (using a non-stick pan) or use polyunsaturated oils such as corn oil, sunflower seed oil, safflower oil, or polyunsaturated soft margarines.

A few words about the inclusion of the above list. Although this book is primarily concerned with obesity and losing weight we should not forget one important reason for losing weight. For many people it is not just to look better but to improve their health and fitness. Arguably, as we saw earlier, by eating a little less of high cholesterol and saturated fat foods you may improve your fitness as a result of decreasing an important risk factor. At the same time you can also save an appreciable number of calories. But it must be emphasized that, unless you have been advised by your doctor to follow a cholesterol-lowering diet for medical reasons, the inclusion of the above list does not imply that you must exclude the foods mentioned. If you enjoy eating them, then continue to eat them. But eat just a little less.

Finally, a 'small print' postscript. Recent research has highlighted the complex nature of the cholesterol question. Although it may be some time yet before definite conclusions are reached, it is now recognized that there are at least three different kinds of cholesterol and other blood fats. These are known as high density, low density and very low density cholesterol and lipoproteins (or HDL, LDL and VLDL, for short). It is thought that high levels of HDL in the blood may remove LDL and VLDL from the walls of blood vessels and so reduce the risk of atheroma formation (and therefore of coronary thrombosis). HDL is thus probably beneficial, whereas LDL and VLDL are probably harmful. Dietary modifications and losing excess weight appear to reduce high levels of LDL and VLDL. Unfortunately diet does not seem to affect HDL, although the evidence suggests that giving up smoking, avoiding excess alcohol and taking regular exercise may increase its level. In the light of current medical knowledge, therefore, it seems sensible to avoid excessive animal fat consumption, to refrain from smoking, to avoid excess alcohol, to take regular exercise – and to keep slim.

7

General fitness

Ask people why they are trying to lose weight and many will answer that, apart from making themselves more attractive, they want to improve their health. In fact what they are also trying to do is to improve their fitness. The distinction is perhaps arguable, but health may be considered to be a state of complete physical, mental and social well-being whereas fitness is the absence of risk factors together with the presence of adequate reserves of vital bodily functions (those of the heart, blood vessels, lungs and muscles). But whatever one calls it – good health or fitness – few slimmers would deny its importance.

Why is fitness important? There are many reasons. First, it creates a feeling of physical well-being and improves stamina. It gives the body reserves of strength essential for strenuous activity and sudden bursts of energy. It allows the body to carry on everyday functions with the least amount of strain on the principal organs and muscle groups. Second, it enlarges our mental awareness and the body's resistance to mental stress. Third, it helps the body to resist physical illness, both major illnesses (such as those of the heart and lungs) and minor ailments (such as colds and sore throats). Fourth, if illness happens, a fit body can cope better with it so that recovery is more likely and more speedy. Fifth, many people feel that if they look better they feel better.

Of course the two groups that make up the concept of fitness – the absence of risk factors together with the presence of adequate reserves of vital bodily functions – are not dissociated. For example, lack of exercise is a risk factor: regular exercise helps to build up the reserves of heart and lung function. So if we examine the risk factors and eliminate them as far as is possible we are simultaneously increasing the body's reserves. What are the risk factors? It would be impossible to describe them all since there are so many. Most forms of self-abuse are risks to our health, for example, smoking, drug addiction, too much alcohol, to name but a few of the more obvious examples. So let us look at some of the more common risk factors.

Being overweight is perhaps the one that most readily springs to mind. As this is dealt with at length in other parts of this book there is no need to discuss it further here. The same applies to lack of exercise which is discussed in Chapter 8. There are three other risk factors which would be usefully discussed here – insufficient sleep, too much stress, and smoking.

Sleep is a mysterious phenomenon which has been the subject of considerable research but about which so much is still unknown. The important point about sleep is that it is a period of tremendous activity. It is the time during which a special hormone called growth hormone is released into the blood stream from a gland called the pituitary which is situated at the base of the brain. The release of the growth hormone is vital for the restoration and repair of all the body's tissues which have undergone considerable wear and tear during our waking hours. This is the reason that someone deprived of sleep has 'bags' under his eyes. Without the essential repair and re-growth our resistance to illness is diminished. The amount of sleep necessary is very variable, some people needing eight or nine hours a night, others much less. But it is not just the length of sleep that is important but its quality. To be of benefit we need to be relaxed when we sleep, which is why, if we are tense or anxious, no matter how long our sleep, we are unrefreshed the next day. Which brings us on to another risk factor – stress.

Stress is also a mysterious concept. It is difficult to define exactly what it is. Further, although stress undoubtedly plays an important part in the causation of disease its precise role is not known. There are two aspects to stress: first, the environmental factors which exert mental pressures on us; and second, our ability to cope with such environmental factors or pressures. If these pressures are too great or our ability to cope with them is inadequate, stress is apparent. Stress manifests itself by the symptoms of anxiety, tension and irritability. As a result, resistance to minor infections is decreased. Perhaps the most significant aspect of stress is its relationship to coronary heart disease. It seems likely that people who live with a lot of stress have a greater predisposition towards heart disease.

Undoubtedly one of the most important risk factors – and hence one of the greatest obstacles to fitness – is smoking.

Smoking

This is probably the best known addictive or dependence-forming use of a drug, the drug being nicotine. By dependence is meant the condition resulting from the interaction between our body and a drug (in this case, nicotine) which has been taken on a periodic, repeated or continuous basis, and causing harm to the person taking the drug and possibly harm to society. These harmful effects may include the compulsion to self-administer a drug the withholding of which causes emotional stress (this being known as psychological dependence); physical discomfort or illness if the drug is withdrawn – in other words, a 'withdrawal syndrome' – (physical dependence); and the necessity for increasing the dose of the drug because of its diminishing effectiveness (known as tolerance). Dependence can occur on many drugs – aspirin, caffeine (as found in tea and coffee), alcohol, the 'hard' drugs (such as heroin, cannabis, LSD and barbiturates) and nicotine (as found in tobacco).

In smoking, nicotine itself plays but a small part in the harmful effects on our physical health. Its danger lies in its addictive qualities which make the smoking habit so difficult to stop once it has become established. Nicotine does not cause much physical dependence but it is undeniably the cause of one of the strongest psychological dependences known. Unfortunately the smoking habit results in some of our most serious diseases.

It is no longer a matter of debate but a matter of indisputable fact that smoking causes disease and kills. Studies have shown that the mortality rate of a smoker is increased by perhaps as much as eighty-four per cent over that of a non-smoker; that the mortality rate increases with the number of cigarettes smoked; that people who start smoking at an early age have an increased mortality rate; and, most encouragingly, that the mortality rate decreases after the habit of smoking ceases. These facts apply to cigarettes but not to cigar or pipe smoking, unless inhalation occurs, when the increased mortality rate is about half that of cigarette smoking.

One problem connected with giving up smoking which is especially relevant to this book is the problem of subsequent weight gain. But it has to be realized that any weight gain is not the direct result of stopping smoking but the effect of eating more – in other words, one addiction (nicotine) is exchanged for another (eating). Although some researchers have claimed that the cessation of smoking increases food absorption from the digestive tract the evidence for this is not convincing and any such increases are too small to be of significance.

The main diseases associated with smoking are those of the heart (coronary heart disease and other cardiovascular disease) and the lungs (cancer, bronchitis and emphysema). There are many other diseases such as peptic ulcers and cancers of the mouth, larynx, gullet and bladder. Although the association between cigarette smoking and disease is a causal one, sceptics argue that the increased susceptibility to disease and the tendency to want to smoke are simultaneously inherited characteristics that have no causal relationship. There are many arguments against their theory, perhaps the best one being that as people stop smoking so the incidence of disease and mortality declines.

Before we look at the main diseases resulting from smoking let us consider for a moment the responsible agents present in tobacco smoke that cause disease. There are three: tar (which contains 'cancer-initiating' and 'cancer-promoting' substances called respectively carcinogens and co-carcinogens), certain gases (especially carbon monoxide) and nicotine.

The mortality from lung cancer is directly related to the number of cigarettes smoked and is between fifteen and thirty times that of a non-smoker. The disease is largely due to tar in the tobacco because of the presence of carcinogens and co-carcinogens.

The mortality from the other major group of lung diseases, chronic bronchitis and emphysema, is also directly related to the number of cigarettes smoked and is about fifteen times that of a non-smoker. Smoking results in a narrowing of the airways which impedes the movement of air in the lungs and which in turn leads to deficient oxygenation of the blood.

Coronary heart disease is the single most common cause of death in the Western civilized world. It causes a third of all male deaths between the ages of thirty-five and sixty-four in the United Kingdom and the United States. Because there are so many different factors in the causation of this disease it is difficult to determine a precise arithmetical relationship between smoking and coronary heart disease, but the increase in mortality is between two and three times that of a non-smoker and tends to be greater in younger smokers. There are two principal factors in smoking in relation to coronary heart disease – nicotine and carbon monoxide.

Nicotine stimulates a pair of glands called the adrenals, situated on the top of each kidney, to secrete substances called catechol-amines into the blood. Catechol-amines increase the stickiness of blood clotting factors called platelets which results in an increased tendency to thrombosis. Further, these substances increase the blood level of fats which results in more fats and lumpy deposits called atheromatous plaques to be formed in the walls of the blood vessels. Catechol-amines also increase the likelihood of abnormalities of heart rhythm which may cause sudden death. In addition, they have other effects which, though not harmful in normal healthy people, may be dangerous in those with narrowed coronary arteries.

The most important aspect of smoking in connection with heart disease is the presence of carbon monoxide in the tobacco smoke. This gas, as a result of competing with oxygen for the receptor sites on the haemoglobin molecule in the red blood cells and forms, instead of oxyhaemoglobin, carboxyhaemoglobin. The resulting under-oxygenation of the blood leads to an increased work-load on the heart and an increased risk of disease and death. Carbon monoxide is the main constituent of old-fashioned town gas. A level of about forty per cent is generally fatal, this being a typical level in those who have died from suicide by gassing. (Natural gas, incidentally, contains no carbon monoxide.) Levels of ten or fifteen per cent are not uncommon in smokers as compared with levels of one per cent in most urban non-smokers. So, by smoking, we are in effect gassing ourselves.

Because it narrows the arteries smoking is an important factor in other diseases of the arteries. For example, if the blood vessels to the brain are diseased by atheroma, smoking may result in further narrowing of these vessels which predisposes to blockage and a possible stroke.

Apart from the diseases already mentioned there is one other major area of concern regarding smoking. This is pregnancy. Smoking causes an increased incidence of prematurity among babies, an increased tendency to miscarry, a greater risk of still-birth or neonatal death, and an increased likelihood to the mother of pre-eclamptic toxaemia (an important condition of which the main manifestation is usually raised blood pressure).

Sadly, there is no easy way to give up smoking. Anti-smoking drugs (of which many different ones have been produced) are generally ineffective. Will-power is really the only successful ingredient in stopping smoking. There are different ways of applying will-power such as reducing by one cigarette each day, delaying the time of lighting up the first cigarette of each day from one day to the next, and going without the cigarettes from which the greatest enjoyment is derived (such as, for example, the cigarette that is smoked after meals). Most people who have given up smoking seem to have done it in the same way – stopping suddenly. This has often resulted from being frightened by the warning signs that they have experienced (such as chest pain due to heart disease). But often, too, it is because they have been motivated by an awareness of the health hazards of smoking. In fact, smoking is a far more serious health hazard than being overweight. But this should not be an excuse for being overweight which still carries significant risks to life. To try to achieve the maximum level of fitness it is important to sleep well, take sufficient exercise, avoid too much animal fat in our diet, drink alcohol in moderation rather

58

than to excess, refrain from smoking, and be of normal weight. This may sound like a counsel of perfection but most people would agree that life is far more enjoyable with a fitter body.

8

Exercise

Most people inevitably think of exercise as a good way of controlling their weight. In fact exercise is not as efficient a way of losing weight as eating less food. For example if you walk one mile at a moderate pace you will burn up the same number of calories as there are in a slice of bread or a cream cracker or 30 grams (1 oz) of plain chocolate. But don't let that depress you because in addition exercise increases your body's metabolic rate which helps to burn up more of the calories that you have eaten.

The main benefit of exercise is that it increases your general level of fitness and probably helps to prevent coronary heart disease, which is more common in overweight people than in others.

How much exercise should I take? This depends on how overweight you are. If you are very overweight you should consult your doctor first, who may suggest that you should take only very mild exercise until you have lost some weight. But if you are only moderately overweight and your general health is good, there is no reason why you should not embark on gentle exercise, gradually increasing in the degree of exertion over a period of weeks. The important point is to avoid sudden or violent exertion which could cause a muscular strain or even a coronary thrombosis, either of which will immobilize you with the result that your weight problem will become even worse!

Should I exercise before or after a meal? Exercise after, rather than before, a meal leads to more food being oxidized to produce heat, and less food is changed into fat which is deposited in the body. So the answer is, exercise *after* a meal is better (but not in the first forty-five minutes whilst your food is being digested).

What sort of exercise should I take? There are endless ways of exercising, but whichever you choose *regularity* is vital. A good brisk walk of twenty to thirty minutes three times a week is far better than a run of an hour or more, or a game of squash, just once a week. New, unaccustomed activities, especially if they are vigorous, can be dangerous and it is generally better to extend existing activities, at least at first. Try to get into the habit of walking faster, using stairs instead of lifts, and walking to the corner shop instead of using the car.

Planned programmes of exercise such as gym 'work-outs', the currently popular aerobics, or jogging, or the sort of exercise that will be described here, should be done only if you are sure that you are in good health and only if you enjoy doing them, otherwise you are unlikely to keep them up with any regularity. Whatever you do, make sure that you break yourself in gently if you are not used to physical activity. Never let yourself become more than *mildly* breathless, and if you experience pain in your chest or if you have a heart condition consult your doctor.

To be of value exercise must fulfil four main aims. These are:

(a) to improve the mobility of your joints

(b) to improve the strength and tone of your muscles, especially those of your back, abdominal wall and thighs. Firm back muscles help to prevent backache; firm abdominal muscles help to get rid of a paunch; and firm thigh muscles improve the shape of your legs

(c) to improve your stamina by increasing the reserves of your heart and lungs

(d) to burn up calories

A planned programme of exercises should start with a few exercises to generally loosen you up and improve the mobility of your joints. These are followed by the muscle-strengthening exercises. Finally comes the exercise to improve your stamina and burn up calories (although of course the first part of your exercise plan will already have contributed to this). There are many excellent books and magazine articles describing such exercises. The ones described here are intended only as a guide. As you should try to exercise every day it is a good idea to try to develop some of your own exercises in order to introduce a constantly changing variety into what can otherwise become a boring chore.

The exercises described below need no special apparatus, will take only a few minutes each day, and can be done in the privacy of your own home or office. But first a few words of caution. If you have any doubt about your general health do consult your own doctor first. Similarly if you are prone to backache ask your doctor about the suitability of the exercises. The number of times you repeat some of the exercises will increase as your fitness improves. But if you have to stop for a few days because of illness remember to 'break yourself in' gently for the first week or two when you resume. At no time should you strain yourself or allow an exercise to give you pain.

Exercise 1 – for loosening up and joint mobility:
Stand upright with your feet 15 inches apart and your arms by your sides. Swing both arms in full circles ten times forwards and ten times backwards. Then repeat.

Exercise 2 – for loosening up and joint mobility:
Stand upright with heels together and slightly raised, toes on the ground, hands on your hips. Keeping your back straight bend your knees slowly so that your trunk is lowered about 18 inches. Return slowly to the standing position. Do this ten times.

Exercise 3 – for loosening up and joint mobility:
Stand upright with your right hand holding on to the back of a chair or a wall for balance. Swing your left leg quite vigorously backwards and forwards while standing on your right leg. Do this ten times and then repeat with your other leg.

Exercise 4 – for loosening up and strengthening the muscles of your back and side abdominal wall:
Stand upright with your feet 15 inches apart and your arms by your sides. Without stooping forwards bend your trunk to your left as far as you can comfortably go, sliding your hand down the outer

side of your left leg. Return slowly to the upright position. Do this five times and then the same to your right side. Then repeat the whole exercise.

Exercise 5 – for loosening up and joint mobility. Also helps a little to strengthen your back muscles:
Stand upright with your feet together and your arms by your sides. Lift your left knee and grasp it with both hands and pull it up and in towards your abdomen and chest. Lower the leg to the floor and repeat with your other leg. Do this ten times.

Exercise 6 – to strengthen your abdominal muscles:
Lie flat on your back on the floor, your legs together and your arms by your sides. Slowly raise both your legs to an angle of 90 degrees, keeping your knees straight, and then slowly lower your legs down to the floor. Do this five times, gradually increasing to ten times.

Exercise 7 – to strengthen your abdominal muscles:
Lie flat on your back on the floor with your feet pressed against a wall or under a heavy chair, your arms by your sides. Slowly raise your trunk to 90 degrees using your abdominal muscles, and then lower again slowly. Keep your legs straight and your feet on the ground. Do this five times, gradually increasing to ten times.

Exercise 8 – to strengthen your abdominal muscles:
Lie flat on your back on the floor, your knees bent, your arms by your sides. Breathe in deeply and slowly using your abdominal muscles, trying to contract them as hard as you can as though you were trying to draw them right into your spine. Then breathe out slowly, pushing your abdominal wall out as far as it will go. Do this ten times.

Exercise 9 – to strengthen the muscles at the sides of your thighs:
Lie on the floor on your left side, supporting your head with your left hand, and with your right arm in front of you with the hand on the floor for balance. Slowly raise your right leg 18 inches, keeping the leg straight, and then slowly lower it. Do this five times, gradually increasing to ten times. Repeat on the other side.

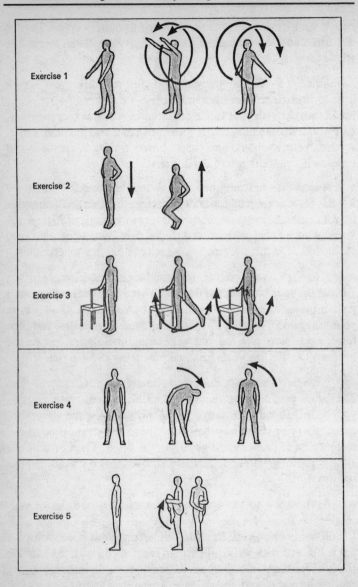

Exercise 1

Exercise 2

Exercise 3

Exercise 4

Exercise 5

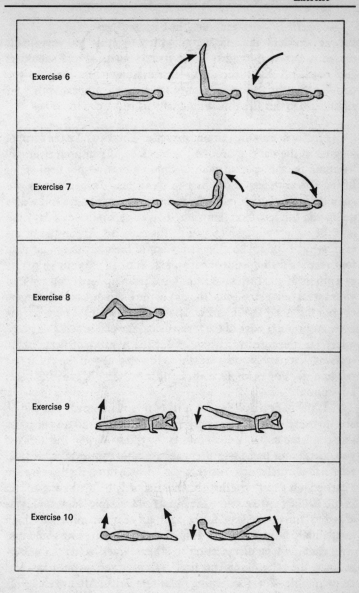

Exercise 6

Exercise 7

Exercise 8

Exercise 9

Exercise 10

Exercise 10 – to strengthen the back muscles:
Lie face down on the floor with your feet together and your hands placed under your thighs. Slowly raise your head and shoulders and your left leg, keeping the knee straight, as high as you comfortably can, and then slowly lower again. Repeat with your right leg. Do this five times, gradually increasing to ten times.

Finally comes the stamina exercise. This can take the form of jogging in the park or around the block or, if you prefer, simply 'running on the spot' at home. Running on the spot consists of lifting alternate feet about four to six inches. To begin with you should not do this for more than a minute. As the days and weeks go by you can lengthen this time (to five or six minutes a day) and also the vigour with which you do the exercise. At the end of the exercise you should be moderately out of breath, but not gasping for breath or feeling faint or nauseated. You can use your pulse rate as a guide. If you turn your right-hand palm upwards you can find your radial pulse by placing the tips of the index and middle fingers of your left hand about an inch above the wrist crease between the bone at the outer edge of the forearm and the pair of tendons in the middle of the forearm. If you count the number of beats in six seconds you merely add a nought to this to give you the pulse rate per minute. For example, eight beats in six seconds is eighty beats per minute.

You will find that as your level of fitness improves you will be able to exercise for increasingly longer periods without your pulse rate going too high. Another interesting thing that you will notice if you check your pulse rate after exercise is that your pulse rate will return to normal much sooner as you become fitter. Some years ago I carried out a test on a British athlete shortly before he was to run in the 10 000 metre event at the Montreal Olympic Games. He was asked to 'run on the spot' fairly vigorously for two minutes (which incidentally he said afterwards he found quite fatiguing compared with running long distances on an athletic track, so do not under-estimate the value of this exercise!). His pre-exercise pulse rate was an incredible 48. (His sleeping pulse rate is 36.) After exercise his pulse rate rose to 72, but returned to normal in less than a minute.

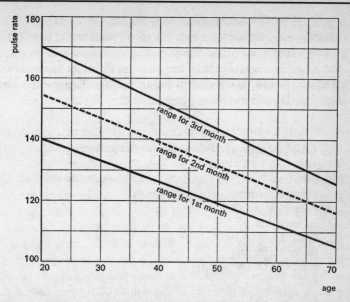

Figure 2. Maximum safe pulse rates according to age and fitness. (Reproduced by kind permission of the Sports Council from *F/40 Fitness on 40 Minutes a Week* by Malcolm Carruthers and Alistair Murray)

Now compare these figures with my own performance after several weeks of inactivity because of illness. My pre-exercise pulse rate was 84. This rose to 164 (definitely not recommended) with exercise and took 27 minutes to return to normal. After one month of regular exercising my exercise pulse rate rose to 144 and took 12 minutes to return to normal. After two months my pre-exercise pulse rate had fallen (another sign of increasing fitness) to 72, rose to 110 on exercise, and took only 4 minutes to return to normal.

One final word about exercise. Try not to look upon it as a chore. Be inventive. Make up new exercises. Involve your family or your friends at work. It is more fun if you do it with other people. In short, enjoy it.

Figure 2 shows the maximum safe pulse rates for people of different ages and different degrees of fitness. It is most important that the rate indicated for your age and fitness is not exceeded. Also if you are in any doubt about your health, or if you are taking tablets prescribed for your heart or blood pressure, it is essential that you consult your doctor first.

A healthy lifestyle will make you fitter. If you are fitter you will be more strongly motivated to losing weight. At the same time losing weight will make you fitter.

TABLE: Calorific values of popular activities

Activity	Calories per minute
sitting or sleeping	1
badminton (singles)	7
cycling (10 m.p.h.)	8
dancing	5
gardening (light)	4
gardening (heavy digging)	8
golf	5
jogging	10
running	14
skipping (rope)	10
squash	10
swimming (33 yds. per min)	7
table tennis	5
tennis (singles)	7
walking (2 m.p.h.)	3
walking (3 m.p.h.)	4·5
walking (4 m.p.h.)	6
walking (upstairs)	20
walking (downstairs)	8

9

Special problems of being a woman

There are three events in a woman's life during or following which obesity is most likely to be a problem: these are puberty, pregnancy and the menopause (or 'change of life').

During puberty the adipose organ (the body fat) enlarges to give the female distribution of fat which gives the characteristic curves and contours to the body. The size of the breasts also increases and this, too, is largely due to the increased deposition of fat. In pregnancy there is considerable weight gain in which an increase in body fat plays an important part.

These effects are largely due to the female hormone, oestrogen, the presence of which is increased at puberty and during pregnancy (until the onset of labour). But this does not explain the obesity which starts at the time of the menopause when oestrogen secretion falls. It may in fact be that as a result of this fall, with consequent tension, depression or possibly even a change in metabolism and decreased efficiency in burning up calories, there is a tendency to eat more food than is needed. It may also be that some women become much less active at this time because their children have grown up and left home. Whatever the reason (or reasons) obesity does seem more common in elderly women than elderly men (although this can partly be explained by the increased prevalence of serious heart and lung disease among men which decreases their chances of reaching old age). Obesity presents a very difficult problem in the post-menopausal woman because the older she is the less easy is it to motivate her. Appealing to her vanity by suggesting that slimness is attractive or fashionable, or appealing to her sense of preservation by pointing out that losing weight may help her to live longer, often have little effect. If she lives on her own and is poor the problem is made worse by the fact that she probably lives on cheap carbohydrate foods which are fattening. She is likely to respond only to sheer enthusiasm and encouragement from relatives and friends.

Mention was made earlier of the importance of oestrogen. One of its effects is fluid retention which causes a temporary increase in weight during pregnancy. But fluid retention as a result of oes-trogen activity occurs in many women every month of their reproductive lives and contributes to the common premenstrual syndrome. Oestrogen causes, in addition to fluid retention, headache, tension, anxiety, depression, cramps, backache, painful breasts and general loss of efficiency. The weight gain (as a result of retained water) can amount to several pounds. This is important to remember when you are slimming because if you do not take it into account you may depress yourself if you compare your weight just after the end of a period with your weight shortly before your next period. This extra fluid (which can also occur when taking the contraceptive pill) is lost during the period itself. But this raises an interesting speculative point with regard to vitamin B. It is claimed by some 'non-Establishment' nutritionists that taking large doses of this vitamin complex can prevent the premenstrual syndrome. In fact, to support this claim there appears to be little or no substantive evidence such as, for example, a clinical trial. But there is a theoretical reason why the claims may have some validity.

Oestrogen is metabolized in the liver where it is converted into weaker derivatives which are themselves broken down and finally excreted in the urine. In the liver oestrogen also increases the activity of an enzyme system necessary for the conversion of an amino-acid, called tryptophan, to nicotinic acid. This conversion requires the presence of vitamin B6, or pyridoxine, and if there are insufficient amounts of this vitamin, there is a disturbance of tryptophan metabolism which is associated with some cases of depression. This depression clears up when large doses of pyridox-ine are given – say, 100 milligrams a day instead of the usual one to two milligrams present in the average diet and usually considered sufficient for most adults. The problem is that pyridoxine deficiency has only been found in a small number of people suffering from depression. But this could be explained by the possibility that some people, especially menstruating women, *may* need more pyridoxine than is presently supposed, perhaps because of some hormonal factor or metabolic change which is too small to measure by currently available methods. This underlines how little we yet know about basic physiology and nutrition and the enormous knowledge that remains to be tapped by advancing scientific technology.

Does this mean that if you are a woman you should take extra vitamin B? In answer, all that can be said at present is that a few women have found that, as a result of taking it, they have passed more urine, thereby diminishing fluid retention. Since it is rapidly excreted by the kidneys you cannot harm yourself by taking too much. So that if you suffer from premenstrual symptoms it may be worth trying, especially as it is readily available from chemists' shops where it can be bought without a doctor's prescription. The essential component is vitamin B6 (pyridoxine) which can be safely taken in doses of 200 milligrams a day. Your chemist can advise you about a suitable preparation containing this vitamin.

10

Overweight children

It may seem odd to devote an entire chapter to the problem of overweight children in a book designed primarily for overweight adults. But there is a very good reason for this. Although some of you may already have grown-up children many of you either still have, or will have, young children or babies. Your eating habits can play an important part in the development of their eating habits. If these eating habits are bad they may become fat. And fat children are unhealthy children.

You may think that very few children are overweight. After all, most babies in these affluent times appear vigorous, healthy, attractive and bonny. Few would disagree, and certainly a vigorous, healthy and attractive baby is desirable. But bonny? Well, what do we really mean by bonny? If you forget that innocent angelic face for one moment and think about a bonny baby quite objectively you will probably agree that by 'bonny' you mean fat. In fact all those bonny baby contests that used to be so popular were designed to favour and reward fat babies – overfed babies.

Recent studies have shown that probably a third, if not more, of all babies in Western civilized countries are overweight in the first year of life. And overweight babies are much more likely to become overweight children than normal babies. And about eighty per cent of overweight children become overweight adults. These overweight adults tend to produce overweight babies. And so it goes on. This is why the problem of overweight children affects most of us at some time in our lives.

Why do babies and children become fat? Although this is such a simple and basic question no one knows the complete answer.

Research papers and the results of studies on the subject appear almost weekly in the medical journals. Their conclusions are confusing, often conflicting, and serve to underline the complexity of the factors involved. In considering this problem there is a remarkably close parallel between the arguments about the cause of obesity and those concerned with the development of intelligence. First, in both obesity and intelligence it has become clear that the first few years of life, even the first months or weeks, are crucial periods. Infant obesity, as has been mentioned, predisposes towards adult obesity. Lack of stimulation in pre-school years may adversely affect the future emotional and intellectual development of a child and even his or her achievements as an adult. Second, controversy about the relative importance of inherited and environmental factors exists in both obesity and intelligence.

Let us look at the causes of baby and childhood obesity and consider first the question of inheritance. Do fat parents produce fat children? To try to answer this it is useful to consider a few statistics. Only about seven per cent of children of parents who are of normal weight are obese. This compares with an obesity rate of forty per cent among children with one overweight parent, and eighty per cent when both parents are overweight. By contrast, the incidence of obesity among children adopted by overweight parents is much less. Studies among identical twins have given interesting results. Such twins, when separated and adopted by different families, tend to retain similar weights to each other and follow much less the weight patterns of members of their adopted families. This is strong evidence that obesity or, what is more pertinent, the tendency to obesity, is at least partly due to inherited factors. But it certainly does not rule out environmental causes. There is strong evidence that many fat parents have fat children because they have 'conditioned' their eating habits badly during the crucial period of infancy. In addition, some older children become fat because they acquire their parents' eating habits. So, having established that childhood obesity is due either to inherited factors or environmental ones or both, let us look at these in more detail.

First, the inherited factors. Weight control depends upon the balance between energy input (food eaten) and energy output (calories burnt up). In Chapter 2 the question of how the body controls the energy input and output 'equation' was discussed in some detail. Briefly, this involves a brain centre that controls appetite – often called the appestat – and a less well understood process that controls body metabolism – something that for pure convenience may be thought of as the 'metabolistat'. It is possible that some children inherit either a defective appestat (so that they eat more than their bodies can burn up) or a defective metabolistat (so that their bodies do not respond to food by burning up calories as efficiently as normal children). This is a simple attractive theory, but the problem is that it is often difficult to determine which is cause and which effect. Although a defective appestat makes a child more likely to overeat, a child born with a normal appestat but who overeats for other reasons may damage his appestat. Similarly, although a defective metabolistat predisposes to obesity – but, please note, does not actually cause it since obesity is the result of overeating – obesity itself may damage the metabolistat.

Other traits which some authorities believe can be inherited are the characteristic of having less food dislikes than most other children (so that more food is eaten) and a 'sweet tooth' (so that sugar and other sweet foods which are very fattening are eaten in excess). A sweet tooth, as we shall see in a moment, may also, and indeed more often does, result from being given sugar regularly during infancy. Another characteristic of fat children is that they tend to move slowly. This applies particularly to the movements that are carried out hundreds of times each day – sitting down, standing up and walking about – so that less calories are burnt up than normal. Of course once a child becomes obese the sheer bulk carried tends to slow him or her down.

What are the other factors, the ones that are not inherited, that play a part in obesity? There are two that are outstanding. The first, which was mentioned briefly earlier, is sugar. Mothers give their babies sugar for many different reasons. Usually it is because it is traditional to give babies sugar – mothers were given sugar as babies by their mothers so why not give their own babies sugar? Also food and drink is fairly unpalatable unless it is sweetened. Or is it? Although it was said earlier that a sweet tooth may be inherited by some children, there is little doubt that the liking for sweet-tasting things is an acquired taste in most children with a sweet tooth. When you think of how so many babies have sugar added to their bottles and added to their drinks this is hardly surprising. And it is all so needless. Apart from providing calories (which are contained in ample amounts in the rest of a baby's natural diet) sugar has absolutely no nutritional value.

The second outstanding factor (that is not inherited) is the early introduction of solids into a baby's diet. Many mothers think that it is of paramount importance to get their babies started on solids as soon as possible. It is as though the late introduction of solids is a sign of retarded development. Unless a baby is genuinely hungry after a milk feed, and that is uncommon before the age of three or four months, there is absolutely no need to start him on solids. Starting solids too soon is likely to make a baby fat.

Does it matter if a baby is bottle- or breast-fed? For thousands of years babies were breast-fed because a baby's mother's milk costs nothing and requires no preparation. Then bottle-feeding became more popular – and it still is. But there is an increasing trend back towards the natural method of feeding. Is this just a fad? Well, apart from its cheapness and ease, breast-feeding has a number of advantages. Breast-fed babies have less tendency to have gastroenteritis – a potentially serious infection of the bowel where diarrhoea and vomiting can cause dehydration. There is also a smaller incidence of atopies – allergies to food: this may be because artificial feeds (which are made from cow's milk) contain many allergy-producing substances called allergens. Breast-fed babies have a smaller tendency to low blood sugar levels – an important cause of fits in babies. Nappy rashes seem to occur less often than in bottle-fed babies. Some authorities believe that the emotional bond between a mother and her baby is likely to be increased by breast-feeding, although there appears to be little actual evidence for this. But most relevant to this book is the fact that breast-fed babies, according to many doctors now, are less likely to become obese. Why this is so is not at all clear. It is known that the composition of human milk changes during the feed so that at the end of the feed there is four or five times as much fat content as at the beginning. It is probable that this is the signal to the baby to stop feeding. It may therefore be an appetite-controlling mechanism. Artificial feeds do not have this change in composition of the milk. It is also possible therefore that in babies deprived of the natural appetite-controlling mechanism of their mother's milk the appestat that was mentioned earlier in this chapter is somehow prevented from developing properly. This may be the reason that babies fed on artificial milk seem to become obese more easily than breast-fed babies, a fact underlined by recent studies which have shown that eighty per cent of bottle-fed babies gain weight faster than optimum from birth, starting with failure to lose weight after birth (such weight loss being the normal occurrence).

Whatever the cause of obesity, fat babies tend to become fat children who, in turn, tend to become fat adults. In addition to the reasons already described, some authorities claim that obesity in the first six months of life leads to an increase in the body's fat cells, not just in size but also in number. The unfortunate child then has to spend the rest of his or her life trying to avoid these extra cells being filled with fat – a difficult and lifelong task.

Some children do not become fat until after infancy, and occasionally not until they are in their teens. One very clear reason for this is lack of exercise. There is unfortunately an increasing trend among children towards sedentary pastimes such as watching television. In schools there is less encouragement to participate in regular sporting activities. Although exercise plays only a minor role in the management of established obesity, lack of exercise is probably a significant factor in the causation of obesity.

Another important cause of childhood obesity lies in the fact that food is a great comforter. In fact some years ago there used to be a popular song about a 'sunshine cake' which illustrates the association that many people have between food and happiness. Children who are unhappy often overeat, and this is usually called compensatory overeating. The unhappiness may result from lack of love and affection at home when the child turns to food as a substitute or else the parents give the child more food instead of the security that the child really needs. A child may overeat because he is small and feels inferior to his friends. By becoming fat and big he tries to overcome his inferiority. Once again there is the problem of which is the cause and which the effect, for although unhappiness may lead to overeating and obesity, a previously happy child, who becomes obese, may become unhappy as a result of being fat.

Remembering that obesity may result not only from a high energy input but also a poor energy output it is not surprising to find that many obese children actually eat *less* than normal children. If they are relatively inactive or if their metabolistats are defective their bodies burn up fewer calories. Normal children can even double their food intake but, because they are active and their metabolism is efficient very little weight will be gained. But even if poor energy output is a major factor in the cause of obesity it cannot be stressed too strongly that it is still overeating that actually *causes* obesity since more calories are being consumed than the body can burn up.

It is sometimes suggested by parents that their child's obesity is due to 'glands'. Let us be quite clear about this. A disorder of the glands or hormones is only very rarely the cause of obesity. In fact most doctors in a lifetime of practice probably never see a single case. A feature of a glandular cause is that the child is usually short, whereas a child who is obese through overeating is of average or above-average height. Clearly if there is any doubt in a parent's mind the child's own doctor should be consulted.

Another common belief is that 'puppy' fat is a normal and acceptable part of childhood and is something that will automatically disappear as a child grows up. In fact, puppy fat is no different from any other kind of body fat and it is the result of overeating. Its presence is not healthy and requires the same positive action as any other kind of obesity.

Does childhood obesity matter? Clearly the answer is yes since most obese children become obese adults and are more likely to suffer the consequences described in Chapter 3. In addition, there are consequences that may occur during childhood. As infants they tend to start walking later and they have an increased risk of having knock-knees and flat feet. And, of course, the delay in walking results in less activity which may further increase the weight problem. Fat children are often more short of breath and are prone to respiratory tract infections. Severe obesity may also affect various organs such as the kidneys.

Now that we have looked at how children become obese, and why it is an important problem, you may then ask what should be done about it. Let us look first at the most important aspect – prevention. The importance of prevention cannot be overemphasized since once a child becomes fat, losing that fat is very difficult.

So often how much a baby eats and weighs turns into a competition with the baby down the road. So, instead of allowing the baby to stop when they have finished sucking, either at the breast or the bottle, they are actively encouraged to have a little more. Each extra half-an-ounce is seen as a triumph by the mother. But a baby does *not* need to finish every drop of every bottle or to suck to the last second of the allotted breast-feed time.

Another common mistake with small babies is offering a milk feed every time the baby cries. Many mums fail to realize that a baby will often cry because of thirst and what is needed is a drink. Do follow advice given at your baby clinic, and if you are not sure which foods to give your baby do not be afraid to ask.

Try not to get into the habit of giving toddlers and children sweets and biscuits on a daily basis, and *never* offer these as a reward for being good. Start good habits of a lifetime by encouraging children to eat fruit rather than crisps and 'junk' food every time they feel hungry. This can be difficult because of the persuasive influence of television, magazines and other children, but it is worthwhile being firm but gentle – *your children's reward will be good teeth, trim bodies and bags of energy*.

Almost all children are vain to a certain extent, and the promise of an attractive body and pearly white teeth without fillings often adds weight to your argument. Also you can wage your own personal war against the media. For instance, in our house, in answer to one TV commercial for a well known, highly calorific chocolate caramel bar, our children sang their own words along with the commercial: 'A — a day helps your teeth rot away!'

Toddlers and small children very often *seem* to eat very little. But, so long as they are healthy, there is no need to worry about their food consumption. The important point is to make sure that they do not binge between meals on chocolate biscuits, sweets, and so on. It is amazing how often a mother will say that her child never eats at mealtimes. But then when you spend some time with the child it soon becomes apparent that the child is eating all the time *except* at mealtimes. Crisps here, sweets there, biscuits here, and so on.

But what do you do with a child who is already fat? Once a child becomes fat it is much more difficult to slim him or her down than it is to prevent the problem from arising in the first place. However, if your problem is that you already have a fat child (and remember that 'puppy' fat is just the same as any other kind of fat!) there is no need to despair. If you follow the basic methods of food preparation in this book you will be helping your child to eat more healthily. The principles of sensible eating are the same whether you are an adult or a child. The only difference is that an overweight adult aims to lose weight, whereas an overweight child should maintain the same weight as growth continues.

Many children love burgers, chips, fish fingers, and so on – 'forbidden' foods in most people's minds. In fact there is no reason at all why children may not eat them, providing this is done sensibly. For example, if possible, grill these foods rather than fry them. Substitute jacket potatoes for chips. Don't fill children up with enormous portions of fattening commercially produced puddings. Give ice-cream addicts small portions, topped with slices of fresh fruit. Don't say no and have an irritable child. Try instead to use your imagination and the ideas in this book to keep you and your offspring happy.

There is little point in giving a separate section of recipes for children in this book because, by and large, children should eat much the same as adults. Instead here is an example of a week's menus for children to provide them with nourishing teatime meals when they come home from school.

| **Monday** | grilled beefburger (100% beef) with jacket potato and wholewheat spaghetti hoops banana and custard |

Tuesday	3 fish fingers with baked beans and a slice of wholemeal bread and low-fat spread *small* portion of ice-cream, served with chopped apple
Wednesday	1 *lean* pork chop, sprinkled with a little sage and onion stuffing, baked in the oven, gas mark 6, 400°F (200°C), for 40 minutes, and served with mashed potatoes and carrots 1 fruit yoghurt
Thursday	Chicken Maryland (see recipe on p. 152) fruit jelly with a *small* portion of ice-cream
Friday	Ham or other cold meat (with the visible fat removed), with a *small* portion of chips and salad (see Chapter 16 for salad ideas) baked apple and custard

Of course the size of the portion cannot be laid down as this depends on many factors, such as the age of the child, whether or not the child is already overweight and, if so, by how much. If the child is not overweight then appetite is a good guide. Some children are blessed with efficient metabolisms which burn up *all* the calories that they consume in excess of their bodies' requirements. If such a child has an enormous appetite, there is nothing to worry about as long as his food is nutritionally sound. Of our own two children one was daily 'dying of terminal starvation' at the end of each schoolday. Sometimes her meal was not ready for when she was about to expire, and so there was always a plate of low-calorie foods ready that she liked, which stopped her from raiding the biscuit tin. Typical foods were a chopped-up carrot, a thinly sliced cucumber, radishes, a green pepper, a slice of melon, or orange slices. These invariably shut her up and kept her happy whilst her main feeding-bag was being prepared.

If you experiment with various foods it is possible to find alternatives to an excess of sticky and sickly sweet things. There are many excellent books on food for babies and children, and if you are really stuck, do consult them. Remember, though, that the same basic rules apply to overweight children as to overweight adults: too much of the wrong kinds of food is what makes people fat. Very often a child's overweight starts in babyhood with an over-anxious mum and continues through to the teenage years when there may develop very unhealthy and unwanted worries about weight which in turn perpetuate bad eating habits that may last a lifetime. Children brought up with good eating habits all through their childhood will have received a cheap but very precious gift that will last them the rest of their lives. It really costs only the time that it takes you to put some thought into what they are eating, and this can even save money on costly chocolate bars, sweets, crisps, not to mention expensive dental bills later.

Unless your child is overweight do not try to ban anything totally as this tends to result in food cravings. The calories from the occasional doughnut or packet of crisps will be quickly burned up by a child of average weight. If your child is overweight it is important to compensate for 'forbidden' foods with low-calorie foods as suggested in the recipes described in this book. Remember that a large bowl of filling and comforting but low-calorie soup can be very helpful, as can puddings prepared in a low-calorie, low saturated fats manner.

There are many schools, even today, which provide stodgy fattening food at lunchtime. It still seems to be a popular idea in such places that it is a virtue for children to eat enormous portions and that it is even more virtuous to have second and even third helpings. You may be unlucky enough to recognize this in your children's school, and you may have noticed that your children put on weight during term that they shed easily during the holiday. If this is so, do campaign at the school for a more sensible and enlightened approach. It may have been sensible long ago in unheated schools, full of undernourished children, to provide highly calorific food. But today there is a far higher percentage of overweight children, and there are very few children who are undernourished.

Of course, some children may be poorly fed in terms of a well-balanced diet but certainly not in terms of calorie intake. Most schools would save time, money and effort if they cut out the pudding course three days a week and replaced it with fresh fruit or a fruit yoghurt. If your children go to a school where either they do not like the food, or you know that the diet is poorly balanced, take advantage of the option (if available) of providing packed lunches. Even a humble sandwich, thoughtfully prepared with good bread and fillings, can be very nutritious (see section on snacks and sandwiches).

A quick word at this point to grandparents. Your grandchildren will still love you – later on, even more – if their treat when they see you is not always a packet of sweets but, perhaps, pennies to be added to their holiday savings. In summer, why not a delicious peach? Even a comic is preferable to sweets every visit.

Finally, in this chapter, a word of caution. It is not my intention to bring up a nation of potential anorectics. Please do not nag your children (unless they are ill because of their excess weight) but, very subtly and gently, try to alter their eating habits without them even realizing it. Children who are going through a slightly podgy stage should not be made to feel freaky or uncomfortable. Rather they should be guided along sensible lines.

Do remember, too, that we are all different shapes. Do not expect everyone to have a Twiggy-like shape, even in childhood. Bone structure dictates the shape of your child's body, and even quite young girls can have fairly pronounced hips without having a weight problem.

11

Can I have some slimming tablets, doctor?

'Can I have some slimming tablets?' is probably the most common question asked of doctors by patients who want to lose weight. Of course it is not always put so directly. Often it is, 'Can I have something to help me slim?' And the patient does not mean a diet sheet or a lecture about eating habits but slimming tablets.

What is the mystique of slimming tablets? What is it about them that can stir up such faith and confidence that would be the envy of any government? What precisely are the magical qualities of these wonder pills that are the slimmer's heaven-sent answer? The mythology surrounding them is quite amazing. But think for a moment about the curious logic – or rather lack of logic – behind them. As we all know, the only way to lose weight is by eating less. This is a basic law of nature, as unbreakable as Newton's law of gravity. What quaint process of reason, then, has led so many people to believe that they can lose weight by eating something extra? Because, after all, whatever you eat and whatever your body absorbs, even the tiniest pill, cannot subtract from your weight (unless it is some kind of 'anti-matter' that cancels out some of the food you eat – a marvellous concept but totally futuristic!). In fact, almost anything you eat, including tablets, is likely to increase your weight. Albeit by only a tiny amount.

To understand the mythology of slimming tablets it is necessary to know exactly what they are and how they are supposed to work. So let us look at some of the different kinds of slimming tablets.

The ones most often prescribed today are *appetite-suppressants*. These used to be drugs such as amphetamine but slightly different ones are now used. However the modern drugs still act in a similar way. They suppress the appetite by acting directly on the body's central nervous system, for it is in part of the nervous system – the hypothalamus – that the centre which controls appetite, the appestat, lies (see Chapter 2). There is no doubt that these drugs are extremely effective in suppressing appetite. But they have a number of drawbacks, some of them being very serious. Because they act by stimulating the nervous system they cause insomnia, irritability and even giddiness in many people. Sometimes people taking such tablets have to have sleeping tablets to help them sleep at night. These drugs can also affect the heart and circulation, causing rapid heartbeat, palpitations and raised blood pressure. There are many other uncomfortable side-effects such as sweating, blurred vision and bowel irritability.

Probably the most serious consequence of this type of slimming tablet is addiction. Addiction is a physical or emotional dependence on a drug. The addictions that most readily spring to mind are those of morphine and heroin. Morphine and heroin are particularly distressing because their withdrawal causes severe physical discomfort and illness (sometimes known as 'cold turkey') due to the strong physical dependence that addicts have on these drugs. Perhaps less obvious examples of addiction are smoking (dependence on nicotine) and alcohol. Here the addict is dependent emotionally on the drug as all those who have tried to give up smoking know only too well! Appetite-suppressants can also lead to a similar emotional dependence. This again is because of their effects on the central nervous system. The stimulation that they can cause may lead to a pleasant sensation of euphoria that becomes an essential part of the slimmer's life. With time the drugs become less effective in producing this euphoria and the number of tablets taken is increased. Eventually the slimmer is unable to live happily without the tablets even if he or she is no longer trying to slim. It may take the same kind of effort to stop taking the tablets as it does to give up smoking. The need to increase the dose of the drug is known as tolerance. As well as emotional dependence a slimmer can develop tolerance to an appetite-suppressant with regard to its ability to diminish appetite. In other words these drugs gradually become less effective.

Another problem with this type of slimming tablet is that if the slimmer successfully loses weight and reaches his desirable weight, stopping the tablets leads to a return of the previous appetite and the inevitable increase in weight once more.

All that has been said does not mean that there is never a place for appetite-suppressant drugs. In severe obesity where there may be medical reasons for wanting rapid weight loss, such tablets may be of use. But such cases form only a minority of overweight people.

The other most commonly prescribed slimming tablet is one that is designed to increase the rate at which the body tissues, especially muscles, use glucose. This drug is said to increase tissue utilization of glucose, which causes the body to burn up more calories than usual, leading to less fat being deposited in the tissues, and so weight is lost. In fact, the evidence that this actually happens does not appear very convincing. Further, it is usually recommended that the slimmer should use the drug in conjunction with a weight-reducing diet. Another theoretical action of this drug is the mobilization of fat from the body's fat stores. Fat that is brought out from these stores is converted to glucose which is then burnt up with the release of calories. Once again, the evidence is not very convincing. Furthermore, apart from some doubt about its efficacy, another problem is that the drug causes a number of side-effects in some people. These usually consist of bowel and stomach upsets, drowsiness and general irritability. Fortunately it does not appear to cause the addiction associated with the amphetamine-type and other appetite-suppressant drugs. Again, like the appetite-suppressants, it has a use, but mainly in the severely obese person.

Most other slimming tablets are highly questionable and nowadays are rarely, if ever, prescribed by doctors. One type of tablet that has been used is a diuretic. Diuretics are drugs that eliminate excess fluid from the body through the kidneys and bladder. They are certainly effective, and quite properly prescribed, in people whose bodies retain an abnormal amount of water as may happen in certain diseases, particularly of the heart. But to try to eliminate water from a fat, but otherwise normal, person is not only ineffective but potentially dangerous. The body has a highly efficient mechanism that carefully controls the water and electrolyte balance of the bodily fluids and the improper use of diuretics can affect this mechanism with the risk of serious consequences. The use of diuretics in slimming was based on the correct observation that fat people often have mild fluid retention. But it is the presence of excess fat, not excess fluid, that makes a person overweight. And it is the excess fat that may be the cause of mild fluid retention. Give a fat person a diuretic and all that happens is that fluid will be lost for a short time, only to return. The fat will not be affected. And to slim effectively it is the excess fat that has to be eliminated.

Hormones used to be another popular kind of slimming tablet and they are still occasionally used in otherwise normal people by quack doctors. (It is stressed by *quack* doctors for, whereas the use of hormones in a person who has a hormone disease and as a possible result is fat may be correct medical treatment, the use of hormones in the absence of a hormone disease is quite wrong. And it must be remembered that hormone disease is an extremely rare cause of obesity.) Hormones are chemical substances manufactured and secreted by certain organs called endocrine or 'ductless' glands. They are called ductless because they secrete their chemicals directly into the blood stream. These chemicals are vital regulators of most of the processes that take place within our bodies. Different hormones have been used, including hormones from the pituitary gland (a small gland at the base of the brain) and sex hormones. They are supposed to mobilize fat from the body's fat depots and although they are still used in the form of injections by some so-called 'obesity specialists' (see Chapter 13) there appears to be little evidence that they are effective, and their use may be dangerous.

Another hormone that used to be popular is thyroxine which is secreted by the thyroid, a gland situated in the neck. This hormone is primarily concerned with controlling the rate of metabolism – chemical processes – in our bodies. A long time ago it was noticed that adults whose thyroid gland produced insufficient thyroxine developed a disease called myxoedema. This disease is characterized by a general slowing down of all the body processes. As a result of this slowing down, the body needs less calories and, unless a person with the disease eats less food, overweight results. By contrast, people with an over-active thyroid gland – a condition called thyrotoxicosis – tend to be lean and over-active. This is because their bodies are burning up more calories than are being consumed. In the light of this it would seem quite logical to take all the fuss out of slimming by simply giving everyone who wanted to lose weight thyroxine tablets. Certainly this is still done in some parts of the world but rarely, if at all, in Britain. The problem is that thyroxine is an extremely powerful hormone which affects very many of the body's processes. In particular, by increasing the rate of metabolism, it can affect the heart and circulation with potentially dangerous consequences.

The same kind of logic led to the use, at one time, of digitalis in slimming. This drug, which is extracted from the foxglove leaf, has been prescribed by doctors for two centuries in the treatment of fluid retention due to heart failure. It increases the efficiency of the heart's pumping action by enabling the heart muscle to use chemical energy more effectively. This led to the belief by some doctors that in a fat, but otherwise normal person, digitalis would increase the heart's pumping action so that blood would be driven round to the tissues much more quickly. In this way the tissues would burn up more energy and the person would lose weight. The fallacy is that digitalis does not improve the efficiency of a normal heart. On the contrary, it may impair the performance of a normal heart and is therefore potentially very dangerous. It must be emphasized, of course, that digitalis (or its modern derivatives such as digoxin) has an important place in the treatment of certain heart conditions and under medical supervision is perfectly safe.

Diabetes is another disease the treatment of which has led to the use of drugs for slimming. People with diabetes have a high blood sugar level. The disease, if acquired in middle or old age, can usually be satisfactorily controlled by diet alone. But sometimes a drug, known as a hypoglycaemic agent, is necessary to lower the blood sugar level. Some doctors have argued that logically the use of such a drug in a non-diabetic fat person will lower the blood sugar level, resulting in the body having to depend on its own glucose and fat stores for energy, with consequent weight loss. This sounds fine in theory, but once again there is little evidence that such drugs are effective in slimming and once more there are potential dangers.

Sedatives and tranquillizers have also been used at various times for slimming. The theory is that the relaxation that results from taking these drugs reduces tension, anxiety and general nervousness which in turn diminishes the appetite. Once again, in the otherwise normal person, there is little evidence that these tablets help to lose weight. It is of course true that some people who suffer from depression or an anxiety state tend to overeat as a result (see Chapter 2). If such a person is prescribed a course of anti-depressant tablets his or her depression may be cured and the overeating, which was merely a symptom of that depression, stops and weight is lost. But depression or anxiety as causes of overeating apply to only a tiny minority of overweight people.

So far all the drugs that have been mentioned are highly active substances that either act on the central nervous system or exert some effect on the body's metabolism. There is another drug – or substance, since it is not really a drug as it is not absorbed into the body from the digestive tract – which is fairly inactive and therefore free of side-effects. This is methylcellulose. It is available either in certain proprietary slimming foods or as slimming tablets. Its effect is quite simple. When swallowed, it absorbs water (which is drunk with it) and swells to fill the stomach and intestines. If this is done before a meal it causes a feeling of bloatedness. It has the added advantage of helping to relieve constipation. The problem is that in spite of the bloated feeling the appetite is usually unaffected. Many doctors feel that bulk substances such as methylcellulose may be of help to a small number of people as a psychological aid to slimming but nothing more.

More slimming tablets available at chemists' shops without prescription are little more than laxatives such as phenolphthalein, aloes or Epsom salts. The theory is that by increasing the activity of the bowel more food is eliminated from the body with resultant weight loss. In fact, by relieving constipation (which they certainly do!) appetite is often stimulated and the would-be slimmer, far from losing weight, may find that weight is gained. There is also a potential danger, particularly if laxatives are used over a long period of time. The muscles of the wall of the intestines may become lax and lose their tone or firmness. The bowel becomes sluggish and there is increased dependence on laxatives for successful bowel action. Furthermore a sluggish bowel may stop working altogether causing an intestinal obstruction which may require a major surgical operation.

Of course laxatives are not usually sold as such for slimming. They are usually 'dressed up' by the addition of other ingredients – usually vitamins, which are unnecessary unless you are eating an unbalanced diet.

So much for slimming tablets. It must be repeated that occasionally there are situations when some of them are justified. But these situations are strictly of a medical nature and occur infrequently. Many doctors feel that for most people slimming tablets are not the best way to try to lose weight. The drugs used may be dangerous or addictive. If weight is lost while taking them, that weight is nearly always put back on again when the tablets are stopped.

12

Slimming diets

There are literally hundreds of diets which appear all the time in books and magazines. In addition there are numerous dieting 'myths'. If one analyses these one sees that they can be classified into a number of broad groups.

1. Diets which are nutritionally acceptable but are likely to leave you feeling hungry, for example, low-calorie diets, low-carbohydrate diets.

2. Diets which are nutritionally acceptable but are likely to leave you feeling hungry and which are monotonous and do not 're-educate' your eating habits, for example, formula diets.

3. Diets which are nutritionally acceptable in the sense that they provide all the essential nutrients, but which contain an unhealthily high proportion of certain nutrients, for example, high fat diets.

4. Diets which are nutritionally unacceptable and are likely to make you feel ill and may cause malnutrition, for example, high protein diets.

5. Dieting myths.

1. Diets which are nutritionally acceptable but which are likely to leave you feeling hungry

These are the low-calorie and low-carbohydrate diets. If followed carefully – in other words by using a diet in a reputable book or magazine – such diets are likely to be well-balanced. The main problem with a fixed diet is that it tends to become monotonous, even if there is a variation for each day of the week. And of course monotony leads to boredom, and boredom to the abandoning of the diet. Also, fixed diets may be difficult to stick to if you have to have your lunch at work (either in the works canteen or office eating your own sandwiches). Alternatively you can work out your own diet each day. The problem then is that you have to carefully calculate and count up the calories or grams of carbohydrate for each meal. This may seem exciting at first but usually soon becomes a chore. There is also a danger that in devising your own menus within a restricted calorie or carbohydrate range, your diet may not be well-balanced.

Another problem, whether you have a fixed or flexible diet, is that to be sure that you are eating only the prescribed amount of calories or carbohydrates you must weigh everything you eat. Many slimming experts dismiss this as nonsense. Yet many people on such diets who have failed to lose weight manage to do so when they start to weigh their food. Their eyes are rather more generous in estimating quantity than their kitchen scales. Even so, weighing your food is a chore to most people. The other main disadvantage of low-calorie and low-carbohydrate diets is that they leave many people feeling hungry. Hunger is an uncomfortable sensation which most people cannot tolerate for long and is the most common reason for the failure of these diets. Also, people with a 'sweet tooth' on low-carbohydrate diets find that their craving for sweet-tasting foods makes their diet difficult to stick to. Another disadvantage of low-carbohydrate diets is that high protein foods are substituted for carbohydrate foods, which makes eating a little more expensive. Also the frequent recommendation which often accompanies low-carbohydrate diets to fill up with foods containing little or no carbohydrate can make losing weight very difficult. The food usually advised is cheese. If you know that 45 grams (1½ oz) of Cheddar cheese contains 180 calories, a similar amount of Stilton 202 calories and 45 grams of cream cheese 348 calories, you would not be too surprised if you found yourself failing to lose weight. Because fats are considered unimportant in such diets there is no restriction on eating fried foods. Yet, for example, the difference between two rashers of fried bacon (170 calories) and a similar amount grilled (80 calories) is 90 calories – equivalent to three teaspoons of sugar.

If, however, you have successfully lost weight on such a diet and if you have kept to your desired weight, do not feel hungry and your general health is good, then keep to it. The chances, of course, are that you are not entirely happy with the diet because otherwise you would be unlikely to be reading this book.

Starvation, in certain circumstances, can be a nutritionally acceptable method of dieting. This does not refer to long-term starvation which should only (if ever at all) be undertaken in hospital under strict medical supervision. What is being referred to is occasional fasting, for example, one day a week or for a few days at a time in a health hydro. The problem is that it does not work to any significant extent. Before some of you protest by saying that you regularly lose weight in this way, let us examine the facts for a moment. As is discussed in Chapter 4, one gram of fat yields about nine calories. This applies to both dietary and body fat. Let us suppose that you are a very active woman. Your daily energy expenditure will be about 2500 calories. If you starve yourself completely for a whole day you will have a negative energy balance of the same 2500 calories. Assuming that in this event your body's energy requirements are met totally by the mobilization and burning up of your body's fat, it is quite simple to calculate how much fat you will lose:

Total calorie expenditure	= 2500 calories
Calorie yield per gram of fat	÷ 9
Fat lost by the body	= 278 grams or 9¾ ounces

The 9¾ ounces is the total amount of fat that will be lost. And remember that this assumes that all the energy is derived solely from body fat. In fact a good deal of it comes also from glycogen (the body's store of carbohydrate) and possibly even from body protein. It is likely that no more than half a pound – possibly much less – of fat will be lost.

So why do some people seem to lose so much weight on even a single day's fasting? The answer is that the bulk of the weight lost is not fat but fluid – water. The reason for this is that a reduction in dietary carbohydrate results in the glycogen store being depleted. Now each gram of glycogen binds three or four grams of water which is excreted by the body. In the first few days of starvation this can amount to two or three pounds of water lost each day. People often resort to starvation after a period of dietary excesses which usually involves the consumption of large quantities of carbohydrates. The accompanying water retention causes the sensation of 'bloatedness', but it is important to remember that people are bloated by fluid, not fat. As is pointed out in Chapter 1, being overweight is the result of too much body fat, not fluid. Any fluid imbalance is soon corrected by the body's efficient regulating mechanisms. So that if you starve yourself after a 'binge' the weight lost will be largely fluid which you would have lost anyway over the following few days. And if you fast after a period of normal eating the weight you lose (again mainly fluid) will soon be regained.

If a real weight loss of a few ounces a day tempts you to starve yourself for several days at a time because simple arithmetic convinces you that a few ounces a day can add up to a few pounds over those several days, such temptation is best resisted. As mentioned earlier, complete starvation can lead not only to the loss of body fat but also body protein – muscle tissue, hormones, enzymes and so forth which is undesirable.

2. Diets which are nutritionally acceptable but leave you hungry and do not re-educate your eating habits

These are of two kinds – the so-called 'one-dimension diets' and the formula diets.

One-dimension diets are so named because they consist largely or exclusively of one food. The best example, and one of the most popular (especially in the United States), is the buttermilk diet. Buttermilk is a somewhat misleading name and sounds as though it should be a cross between milk and butter, and delicious too. It actually gets its name from the fact that it is the waste product of butter manufacture. It is milk which contains no fat – in fact, it is very similar to skimmed milk (milk that has had all its cream skimmed off and thus contains no fat) only more acid. Milk, and therefore buttermilk, too, is highly nutritious, as you would expect from the fact that most young animals (including many human babies) are fed entirely and exclusively on their mothers' milk. It is in fact Nature's most nutritious single food. It contains all the groups of nutrients – proteins, fats, carbohydrates, minerals, vitamins and water. Buttermilk (and, of course, skimmed milk) is even healthier since it contains little fat and therefore its cholesterol and saturated fatty-acid content is low. The buttermilk diet usually entails drinking about six glasses of milk, spaced out at intervals, each day. Because milk is somewhat deficient in iron and vitamins C and D, these have to be taken as tablets each day. An unlimited amount of liquid (including tea and coffee) is allowed so long as it contains no calories. No sugar is allowed. Low-calorie drinks are also allowed.

A similar one-dimension diet is the yoghurt diet. Yoghurt is made from milk (usually skimmed) by curdling with special bacteria. Again it is very nutritious but if it is the only food eaten added iron and vitamins are essential.

There are variations of these diets – for example, buttermilk and cottage cheese and buttermilk and bananas. There are of course many other one-dimension diets but since these consist of foods other than milk – for example, vegetables only or fruit only or fruit and vegetables only – they lack many essential nutrients and are unhealthy.

Formula diets are extremely popular. They are in effect substitute meals for they contain all the nutrients that our bodies need. They may come in the form of liquid or powder to which water is added or biscuits. They have a known quantity of calories. For example, the currently popular very low-calorie diets, such as the Cambridge and Modifast diets, provide about 400 calories a day. The fact that formula diets contain all the essential nutrients, require little or no preparation and obviate the need to plan meals, makes them very attractive – at first. After a time the sheer monotony of such a diet leads to boredom, and boredom sounds the death-knell for any diet. Also, because many of them contain little bulk, constipation often becomes a problem, although some formula diets partially overcome this difficulty by having added methylcellulose. The overwhelming disadvantage of such diets is the fact that they break one of the most important rules of sensible dieting – they do not encourage you to re-educate your eating habits. Inevitably the time will come when you will want to stop using the formula diet, either because you have reached your desirable weight or because you are simply bored with the diet, and then you are likely to return to your old eating habits and put weight back on again. However, for some patients needing to lose a lot of weight quickly, the short-term use of very low-calorie diets may be useful.

3. Diets which provide all the essential nutrients but are nevertheless unhealthy

The best example of such a diet is the high fat diet. The principle of this diet is that carbohydrates are virtually eliminated from the food. The problem is that most fat we eat is animal fat because the choice of vegetable fats is quite limited (safflower oil, sunflower oil, soya-bean oil, for example). Animal fat, as we saw in Chapter 6, contains a lot of saturated fatty-acids. And there is a strong correlation between high saturated fatty-acid intake, blood cholesterol and heart disease (all of which is discussed in Chapter 6). So in the light of current medical evidence it is difficult to justify the use of such a diet.

4. Nutritionally unacceptable diets

These are the diets which, if you can manage to stick to them, will undoubtedly lead to loss of weight – often dramatically. They are also likely to lead to severe malnutrition – usually not so dramatically, but none the less seriously. Such diets are legion.

High protein (or even all protein) diets are among the most popular of these fad slimming diets. I am referring to those in which you eat as much meat, fish, eggs and so on as you like but little or no carbohydrate. They are nutritionally unacceptable for two main reasons. First, the processes by which the body uses amino-acids (the basic units that make proteins) require a lot of water. A high protein diet can lead to serious fluid imbalances. Second, a diet lacking in carbohydrates inhibits the body's utilization of protein in protein's important roles of growth, tissue repair, hormone synthesis, and so forth. As a result the amino-acids are broken down and many of their constituents are excreted by the kidneys. (Some doctors believe that after a time such diets can lead to impairment of kidney function and possibly even permanent damage.) Let us look for a moment at this 'protein-sparing' function of carbohydrates.

Carbohydrates, being high in calories, are our bodies' most important source of energy. Glucose is quickly and efficiently burnt up to release this energy. The presence of carbohydrates therefore allows the amino-acids derived from proteins to be used for their main function of tissue growth and repair. Some nutritionists believe that there is another explanation for carbohydrate's protein-sparing action. It is known that amino-acids (the end-products of protein digestion) after being absorbed from the digestive tract are carried in the blood to the liver. Here they enter the 'amino-acid pool' and their subsequent fate depends on the presence or absence of glucose. In the absence of glucose, liver enzymes (called 'deaminases') break up the amino-acid groups into nitrogen (which is converted into urea and excreted by the kidneys) and a residue. This residue, which consists of carbon, hydrogen and oxygen, is converted either to glucose (which is burnt to release energy) or fatty-acids, depending on the amino-acid. Thus the amino-acids are used as fuel. But if glucose is present, the amino-acids are not broken down. It is thought that glucose may actually inhibit the breaking-down process by inhibiting the deaminases.

A typical high or all protein diet is one which prohibits all food except lean meat. Other diets allow only fish. And some diets allow only eggs – particularly unhealthy since eggs are such a rich source of cholesterol which most doctors now agree should not be eaten in excess. Apart from their expense and monotony such diets can make you ill. After only a few days you are likely to have bowel disturbances and you may feel tired and generally 'off-colour'. Over a longer period of time there is the very real risk of severe malnutrition.

5. Dietary myths and fallacies concerned with slimming

There are literally hundreds of old wives' tales concerned with dieting in order to lose weight. Although they are sheer nonsense it is worthwhile, not to say interesting and perhaps even amusing, to consider just a few of the more popular ones.

The most common fallacies are those concerned with water. In fact, water has acquired quite a mythology of its own. Sometimes the advice given to a slimmer is to drink more water than usual. Apparently this is supposed to 'flush out the system'. Precisely which system is supposed to be flushed out and why it is particularly important for slimmers is a curiously elusive piece of information. It may be a case of a little knowledge being a dangerous thing, for patients with cystitis (infection of the bladder) are advised, quite correctly, to increase their fluid intake. This is to 'flush out the system', but for cystitis sufferers, unlike slimmers, this is not just a vague and meaningless expression. The system concerned is the urinary system, and what is flushed out are the infecting organisms – the bacteria.

Some slimmers are advised to drink a glass of water before each meal. This is in the mistaken belief that by so doing they fill up their stomachs with water and so they will feel full and will eat less.

Other people are given the opposite advice. Rather than drink more water they are told to drink less water – or even none at all. A typical statement is that it is bad to drink water with a meal, and so fluids should be drunk only *between* meals. Again it is difficult to understand the rationale for this kind of advice. Other people say that water dilutes the gastric juices and is therefore bad for digestion. Of course this is nonsense. Other people think that water is fattening. Again this is quite untrue since water contains not a single calorie. Advice about water restriction can be harmful because if the body is deprived of too much fluid it becomes dehydrated. Over a long period of time this could lead to the formation of stones in the kidneys and recurrent infections of the urinary system.

Severe water restriction can disturb the body's metabolism as can salt restriction – another piece of advice sometimes given to slimmers. Certainly the presence of a lot of salt in the body attracts a lot of water with a tendency to water retention. But it is not water that makes people fat, but fat. In any case if an excessive amount of salt is eaten the resulting water retention is only temporary as the body has a highly efficient regulating mechanism which ensures a correct fluid balance. Lack of salt can cause serious consequences. In very hot weather your body sweats profusely and a lot of salt is lost. If you drink large amounts of water – as you are likely to do because of thirst – and you do not take any extra salt, you may become ill and weak because of salt depletion, a condition commonly known as heat stroke. Apart from the dangerous consequences of salt restriction, whether in hot weather or in normal conditions, lack of salt in your diet makes your food rather unappetizing. Some would answer that that cannot be bad since then you are likely to eat less! This is true but, as was said earlier, the medical consequences can be serious and in any case an unappetizing diet is one that you are unlikely to stick to for long.

Some slimmers believe that vitamin pills have magical weight-reducing powers. Whether this notion is fed to or derived from the fact that some so-called slimming tablets that can be readily bought in some chemist and health food shops contain little more than simple vitamins is not clear. Of course vitamins have absolutely no effect on whether or not you lose weight. If you are on a crash diet you may well need vitamins because these are missing from your food. But if you are on a well-balanced diet, there is no need at all for extra vitamins.

The 'grapefruit diet' is an old favourite that never seems to go out of fashion. There are many variations of this but the most common form it takes is the eating of half a grapefruit at the start of every meal. The theory is that grapefruit has the property of converting fat into energy. There is absolutely no evidence that this is so. Of course grapefruit contains very few calories and is therefore not very fattening itself. Perhaps the reason it seems to work for some people is that those people are very weight-conscious and make a practice of generally eating less food.

13

Other slimming methods

This chapter will describe some of the methods, clubs, clinics and so on that aim to help people in their weight-control programme. They vary enormously in their effectiveness, some being very good whereas others are quite useless. Some are cheap, others are expensive. More important, whereas some are harmless others can be very dangerous. Remember, too, that a method which suits one person may not be suitable for another.

Dieting methods will not be discussed as these are described in Chapter 12. No mention will be made of slimming tablets (see Chapter 11) or exercise in general (see Chapter 8) although clubs and exercising gadgets will be mentioned.

It is impossible to include all the available slimming methods and aids as there are so many of them. But we can look at some of the most popular ones.

Group slimming clubs

The stimulus of joining a group of fellow slimmers, paying for the privilege, badges for success, public shame for failure are features which have made slimming groups very popular. All of them require strict dietary restrictions which in many cases, such as Weight Watchers and the Silhouette Slimming Club, are medically sound. The problem with their diets is that they generally require substantial changes in your choice of food which, as is explained in Chapters 12 and 14, can be difficult to persevere with in the long term. Undoubtedly there are successes but the failure rate does seem rather high. It is also an unhappy fact that there are some less well-known group slimming clubs which use medically unsound diets such as a high protein combined with very low carbohydrate diet. Any group of people can join together and form their own slimming club, and many such isolated clubs exist, but ultimately they are only as successful as their dieting methods which are not always the best. Of course, if you are successfully losing weight by belonging to a reputable club there is no need for you to stop.

Slimming clinics

These are commercial establishments where, for what is often a large fee, you will be offered a weight-reducing programme consisting of treatment with an artificial exercise machine, electric vibrator belt and similar apparatus – and a diet. Successful weight loss depends solely on the diet, a fact which is sometimes glossed over by such clinics.

Health hydros

These offer a most pleasant way of losing weight in congenial surroundings and at a price. What many people fail to realize, however, is that much of the weight loss (which can be as much as five or six pounds a week) is water rather than fat. As is explained in Chapter 11, starvation (or a diet very low in carbohydrates) leads to the utilization of the body's store of carbohydrate which, as it binds water, causes water to be eliminated from the body. Water is rapidly regained by the body when the period of starvation is ended. The other problem about strict dieting is that eating habits are not re-educated which is a further reason that many people quickly regain their weight after leaving a health hydro. On the other hand, other benefits are undeniable, especially the relaxation and general feeling of well-being resulting from the rest, massage treatments, saunas and other special baths. If you can afford it a health hydro is probably a much healthier place at which to stay for a holiday than a five-star hotel. But do not be fooled by the weight loss.

Saunas and Turkish baths

Once again, a pleasant way of passing the time of day, and one that promotes (for a short time) a general feeling of well-being. But it has to be remembered that the weight lost through sweating is not fat but water which is very quickly replaced.

Exercise clubs

As is explained in Chapter 8, exercise by itself is most unlikely to lead to weight loss. Providing that you remember this, exercise clubs offer superb equipment (which can be a great psychological stimulus) for exercise which is undeniably important for your general health and which, if done *in conjunction with eating less*, can help you in your weight-control programme. But of course you can exercise perfectly adequately in your own home without any special apparatus (see Chapter 8).

Exercise machines and gadgets

These are legion and different ones seem to be in fashion at different times. Examples are rowing machines, bicycling machines, chest expanders, weights, and various gadgets using ropes and pulleys. Again they provide useful incentives to exercise but you must not forget that you must also eat less if you are to lose weight. Remember, too, that to be of value exercise must help you in one or more of four aims – to improve the mobility of your joints, to improve the strength of your muscles, to improve your stamina by increasing the efficiency of your heart and lungs, and to use up energy. In evaluating the usefulness of any piece of apparatus apply these aims and see how many are fulfilled. And, of course, no form of exercise will be of benefit unless it is done regularly, for example, every day or two to three times a week.

Spot reducers

Once again, these are legion. They are based on the fallacy that you can lose weight from selected areas (such as your thighs) without losing weight from other parts of your body. There are even clinics which offer to rid you of something called 'cellulite' which is supposed to be lumpy deposits of fat due to water-logged toxin-infested fat cells, although there seems to be little evidence for its existence.

Some of the machines work on the principle of breaking down fat cells, for example, massage machines and vibrator belts. In fact, unless you eat less, there is no appreciable fat loss: and if you do eat less you are unlikely to lose more fat from the areas to which the machine has been applied than other parts of your body. Other machines work by electrical stimulation of groups of muscles causing them to contract. There is no doubt that they do improve the strength and tone of the muscles but the machines are very expensive and you can achieve the same result by exercising with the added benefit of using up energy. These machines, which are in use in slimming clinics, health hydros and physiotherapy departments, are probably most useful for people who are not fit enough to exercise. Various types of garments – corsets and inflatable belts, for example – are also claimed to help in spot reduction by making you sweat. Of course, all you lose is water, not fat.

Hypnotherapy

Hypnosis and psychotherapy are used to help some people to lose weight. The results can be very good, but only in patients who are strongly motivated towards losing weight.

Injections

For some years claims have been made that regular (usually daily) injections of chorionic gonadotrophin (a hormone obtained from the urine of pregnant women) are effective weight reducers. It has been shown, however, that injections of water are probably equally effective, providing the patient is not aware that the injected substance is simply water and that he (or she) is on the same low-calorie diet which patients having injections are usually given (and which is probably the real cause of any weight loss). Quite apart from whether or not such injections do help you to lose weight the use of hormones as a treatment for obesity is thought by some doctors to be potentially dangerous.

Surgery

This is the last resort and is reserved for the grossly obese patient who, generally for psychological reasons, is quite unable to lose weight. A variety of operations have been devised. The simplest is the removal of large wads of fat from various parts of the body, especially the abdominal wall (an operation aptly known as 'apronectomy'), but also from the breasts, arms and thighs. It is entirely a cosmetic operation principally designed to give the patient a morale boost. Unless it is followed by dietary measures the fat quickly returns.

Jaw-wiring is a technique which prevents the patient eating solids. The patient lives on a low-calorie fluid diet with vitamin and iron supplements.

There are major operations designed to interfere with the digestion and absorption of food. One involves the removal of ninety per cent of the stomach, but this is a difficult operation technically in a very obese person. Another procedure involves by-passing much of the small bowel – the jejunum and ileum – where most of our food is absorbed. Good results have been claimed, patients losing on average more than a third of their original body weight. The problem is that there is a high mortality rate (as much as five per cent) either as a direct result of surgery or subsequent complications such as liver failure or coronary thrombosis. Apart from mortality many patients suffer distressing side-effects resulting in the necessity to reverse the operation.

Having now considered some of the non-dietary aids to losing weight let us remember once again that the only way to lose weight is to eat less.

14

How to lose weight without really dieting

So far in this book obesity has been discussed from the point of view of what it is, what causes it, and why we should do something about it. Some of the popular slimming methods have been described and why these are often disappointing. Now we can look at how to lose weight successfully.

Because the successful application of any method (whether it be concerned with losing weight, driving a motor-car or taking good photographs) requires a firm understanding of the whys and wherefores of that method, it is necessary to consider first the essentials of a successful slimming method. Briefly these are:

   (i) Weight must be lost

  (ii) Weight lost must not be regained

 (iii) The period of losing weight must not be accompanied by distressing symptoms (such as hunger)

 (iv) The food must contain all the necessary nutrients

  (v) Losing weight must not become an antisocial process

 (vi) Losing weight must be a pleasant process

(vii) Losing weight must be a simple process – it should not be physically or mentally taxing

Let us look at each of these criteria in more detail.

(i) Weight must be lost

This may seem an absurdly obvious statement but there are many slimming methods which do *not* lead to weight loss. This may be due to a fault in the method or incorrect application of the method.

As an example there are many people who put themselves on a

1000-calorie diet (a popular weight-reducing diet) and are puzzled when they find that they do not lose weight. This leads them to reduce their calorie intake from 1000 calories a day to 800, then to 600, and finally to 400 calories – with no weight loss! They remain completely mystified by their failure to lose weight. But if they subsequently weigh their food and keep an accurate diary of what is eaten they find that even on the supposed 400-calorie diet they are in fact eating as much as 1600 calories each day. Their servings are generous, to say the least!

This illustrates that no matter how faithfully you follow a diet (or think you do) unless you actually lose weight it is all a waste of time and effort.

(ii) Weight lost must not be regained

Few people would deny that losing weight is a pointless exercise if all the weight lost is subsequently regained. Yet so many slimmers do precisely that. In fact, it is probable that the majority of people who diet return to their previous weight. The reasons for this are not hard to find. 'Crash diets' are the worst culprits. They involve some degree of starvation with inevitable hunger. Hunger is a distressing sensation and few people can put up with it for any length of time. So, although weight is rapidly lost, the diet is not followed for long, with a consequent return to the would-be slimmer's previous eating habits. All those pounds which looked so beautiful during their departure are decidedly less attractive during their return. To make matters worse, the unsuccessful slimmer loses heart to such an extent that he (or she) not only returns to the previous weight but often exceeds it. There is an additional problem that the psychological effect of having failed once makes a person less likely to try again in the future.

Of course it is not only 'crash diets' which create these problems. Any weight-reducing diet or slimming aid which, in the course of time, creates a situation in which weight lost is regained is bad.

(iii) Losing weight must not be accompanied by distressing symptoms

Hunger is the commonest reason for the failure of weight-reducing diets. This distressing sensation causes mental symptoms (irritability, anxiety, nervous tension, depression) and physical symptoms (headaches, drowsiness, fatigue). The slimmer's relationships with relatives become strained, as do those with friends and workmates. It is merely a question of time before the diet is abandoned.

(iv) The food must contain all the necessary nutrients

Since, for many people, one aim of losing weight is to promote health and well-being the diet must contain all the necessary nutrients – otherwise malnutrition may result with consequent deterioration of health. Fad diets and 'crash diets' are notorious examples of the type of diet which excludes many essential nutrients.

(v) Losing weight must not become an antisocial process

Most of us have had the experience of inviting a friend to dinner which has been prepared with loving care – not to mention the expense and time – only to find the food being rejected with the excuse, 'I'm on a diet. It smells absolutely delicious but I'm not allowed to eat it – it's much too fattening.' Yet so many diets require the kind of discipline to refuse appetizing food. Such diets are impractical because they make eating in a restaurant or a works canteen, or indeed anywhere apart from at home, quite impossible. And they are completely unnecessary. Losing weight – and keeping to an ideal weight – should be a permanent state of affairs. So if losing weight means not being able to eat out, then losing weight is being done in the wrong way.

(vi) Losing weight must be a pleasant process

Quite apart from the problems of hunger and diets lacking in essential nutrients, if losing weight means having to go without all your favourite foods – or eating mainly foods that you do not like – you are unlikely to persevere with your diet. Losing weight must be a pleasant process or it will not succeed.

(vii) Losing weight must be a simple process

Even in these days of pocket-calculators, diets which require constant weighing of servings or thrice-daily calculations of calorie or carbohydrate unit intake are a chore. Such a chore is both mentally and physically exhausting. Deciding what and how much food you are going to eat each day must be a simple process.

So where does that leave us? Well, you might be forgiven for thinking that losing weight successfully, if all the above criteria are to be satisfied, is surely impossible.

But there *is* a way to lose weight – successfully. It is based on two very important principles. And it is absolutely essential that these principles are known and understood.

The first principle is this. Losing weight is not a question of 'going on a diet' or 'following a diet' or anything whatsoever to do with 'diets'. Losing weight is a question of *re-educating your entire eating habits*. And, as you will see in a moment, that is not nearly so drastic as it may sound.

The second principle is just as basic. Losing weight must be done *slowly*. This is something that just cannot be emphasized too strongly. Weight must be lost slowly. Weight that is lost quickly is weight that is almost always put back on again. Weight that is lost slowly is weight that is usually lost permanently.

But what is meant by slowly? There is no single answer to that question. What may be slow for one person may be fast for another. But in general what is meant is a mere one or two pounds a week – certainly no more. In some cases weight loss should be even less – perhaps only half a pound a week. You may think that you will never get down to your desirable weight like that. Well, let us look at an example. Suppose that you are two stones (twenty-eight pounds) overweight. A weight loss of two pounds a week will bring you down to your desirable weight in fourteen weeks – just over three months: a weight loss of one pound a week in six months. And that is really very little time indeed, especially when you consider all the time it takes to lose weight with strict conventional diets, when you then lose heart, pile all the weight back on again, and then start all over again. Many people spend years, maybe even a lifetime, trying to lose weight, unsuccessfully.

The two principles that have been described – re-educating your eating habits and losing weight slowly – are not entirely separate. In fact, they have a common link. The link is the actual method by which you lose weight.

To lose weight all you need to do is to *eat a little less*. Just a little less, please note, not a lot less. Two potatoes instead of three. One slice of toast instead of two. Two beers instead of three. Every time you eat, eat just a little less. With two exceptions (which will be described in a moment), do not change the food you eat or the drinks you drink. Never mind if people tell you that that piece of cake or that bar of chocolate is full of calories. If you like the cake or the chocolate then eat it – only have a *little* less than you would have done previously.

The two exceptions to the basic principle that you do not need to change your food are these: first, whenever possible use a less fattening method of cooking. For example, grill your bacon instead of frying it. You can save 80 to 100 calories per portion and most of you will agree that there is little difference in the taste: in fact, many people find grilled food more pleasant because it is less greasy. If you do need to fry use a non-stick pan and fry in the food's own fat. In this way you can save 40 calories in a fried egg. With minced meat dishes do not pre-fry vegetables in oil or fat but first heat the meat slowly and fry it in its own fat. Then add your vegetables. There are other cooking 'dodges' that do not materially alter the taste of the food. For example, do not thicken gravy with flour. This applies, for instance, with steak-and-kidney pies when you could go further by avoiding a double crust – just have a single crust on top.

The second exception to the basic principle needs very little thought. Never use sugar. Each teaspoon contains about 30 calories. Either 'train' yourself away from your sweet tooth or use artificial sweeteners which are available in tablet, liquid and powder forms. If you want a sweet taste with your cornflakes or pancakes use artificial sweetening powder which contains no calories. Similarly with your tea or coffee use sweetening tablets. And it is surprising how many cooked sweet foods are very palatable when artificial sweeteners are used. Use low-calorie soft drinks. Two ounces of ordinary squash concentrate contain 70 to 80 calories: the same quantity of low-calorie squash has about three calories. And most people can hardly taste the difference. In fact many people find that a slimline tonic water (about one calorie per can) is more refreshing than ordinary tonic water (about 90 calories per can).

You will probably agree that the two 'exceptions' described do not materially change the food and drink that you consume since the taste remains largely the same and possibly even improved. But you will save a lot of calories. And this is in addition to the basic principle of just eating less. All those tiny little bits of food that you are not eating add up to weight that you are going to lose. Only a small amount of weight, true, but over a period of a few weeks or a few months enough to bring you down to your desirable weight. At the same time as you have been losing weight slowly you have been re-educating your eating habits: because in a very short time you will find that you no longer have to make a conscious effort to eat less. And as your eating habits have been re-educated you are unlikely to pile all that weight back on again.

As an illustration – and to answer the sceptics amongst you – some typical meals will be described to show how you can save calories with very little effort. It must be emphasized, however, that it is not necessary for *you* to do this. The calories are being counted simply to *demonstrate* how the principle of eating a little less works. For convenience, calorific values will be quoted in round figures.

Let us start with breakfast. The first course is cornflakes:

Cornflakes	typical portion:	
	30 g (1 oz)	100 calories
+ milk	typical portion:	
	140 g (5 oz)	95 calories
+ sugar	typical portion:	
	10 g (2 tspns)	60 calories

Total	255 calories

Now let us see what happens if we reduce the size of the portions by just a little:

Cornflakes	20 g (⅔ oz)	70 calories
+ milk	85 g (3 oz)	55 calories
+ sugar	5 g (1 tspn)	30 calories

Total	155 calories

Now let us see what happens if we substitute low-calorie foods where possible:

Cornflakes	20 g (⅔ oz)	70 calories
+ skimmed milk	85 g (3 oz)	30 calories
+ artificial sweetener		0 calories

Total	100 calories

So, by reducing the size of the portions we have saved 100 calories. And by using low-calorie substitutes we have saved a further 55 calories – a total of 155 calories saved on just one course. Of course you may not want to use skimmed milk (a surprisingly easy taste to acquire, incidentally) so that if you continue to use whole milk you can still save 130 calories overall.

Instead of cornflakes (or as well as) you may prefer to start with the traditional bacon and eggs:

Bacon (streaky), fried	2 rashers	170 calories
Egg fried in butter or oil	one	135 calories
Total		**305 calories**

Smaller portions:

Bacon, fried	1 rasher	85 calories
Egg fried in butter or oil	one	135 calories
Total		**220 calories**

Now if we grill the bacon and fry the egg in its own fat in a non-stick pan:

Bacon, grilled	1 rasher	40 calories
Egg fried in its own fat	one	95 calories
Total		**135 calories**

So we have saved 85 calories by eating less bacon and a further 85 calories by grilling the bacon and dispensing with fat for frying the egg – a total saving of 170 calories. And the bacon will be crisper.

Now for toast and marmalade. (Incidentally toasted bread has no fewer calories than untoasted.)

Toast	2 slices	145 calories
Butter (½ oz per slice)	30 g (1 oz)	225 calories
Marmalade (½ oz per slice)	30 g (1 oz)	75 calories
Total		**445 calories**

If we have just one slice of toast and spread the butter and marmalade more thinly:

Toast	1 slice	70 calories
Butter (¼ oz per slice)	7 g (¼ oz)	55 calories
Marmalade (¼ oz per slice)	7 g (¼ oz)	20 calories
Total		145 calories

Substituting low-calorie equivalents where possible:

Toast	1 slice	70 calories
Low calorie margarine	7 g (¼ oz)	25 calories
Low calorie marmalade	7 g (¼ oz)	10 calories
Total		105 calories

We have saved 300 calories by eating less toast and spreading thinner layers of butter and marmalade and a further 40 calories by using low-calorie margarine (the difference in taste of which you will barely notice sandwiched between toast and marmalade) and low-calorie marmalade.

Now for the coffee:

Coffee	85 g (3 oz)	(3 calories)
+ milk	85 g (3 oz)	55 calories
+ sugar	10 g (2 tspns)	60 calories
Total		115 calories

A smaller cupful (4 oz instead of 6 oz):

Coffee	55 g (2 oz)	(2 calories)
+ milk	55 g (2 oz)	40 calories
+ sugar	5 g (1 tpsn)	30 calories
Total		70 calories

Using low-calorie substitutes:

Coffee	55 g (2 oz)	(2 calories)
+ skimmed milk	55 g (2 oz)	20 calories
+ artificial sweetener		0 calories
Total		20 calories

We have reduced one cup of coffee by 45 calories simply by drinking less, and by a further 50 calories using low-calorie equivalents. In the whole breakfast (if you were to have all four courses which would constitute a very hearty breakfast) you would have reduced the original total of 950 calories to 550 calories by just eating a little less (a saving of 400 calories), and to 465 calories by not frying in fat (a saving of 85 calories), and to a final 340 calories by using low-calorie substitutes (saving a further 125 calories) which is a total saving of 610 calories. There is an added bonus in that by avoiding frying and using less butter or margarine, less saturated fatty-acids are eaten with probable benefits to your health (see Chapter 6).

Now the mid-morning snack. Again, a cup of coffee can be reduced, as we have seen, from 115 calories to 20 calories. Suppose you also have two chocolate biscuits which may amount to a further 170 calories. By having just one biscuit you save 85 calories. Alternatively, unless you have a particular penchant for chocolate biscuits, you may be just as happy with a morning coffee biscuit which costs you only 25 calories. This illustrates two important points. First, eating less of some foods is going to help you more than eating less of other foods. Although you do not have to worry about the different kinds of foods if you are just generally eating less, it clearly helps if you eat even less of the really fattening foods (such as chocolates and sweets) than those foods which have few calories (such as green and salad vegetables). But it must be stressed that you do not have to eliminate chocolates and sweets from your food if you really enjoy them. Which brings us to the second point. Sweet-tasting foods are eaten almost entirely for their taste. For example, suppose that you happen to love home-made vanilla chocolate truffles. Whereas you used to eat two or three at a time try instead sharing *one* with perhaps your husband or wife. Bite off a tiny piece at a time, chew it slowly and savour its flavour for as long as possible before biting off the next tiny piece. That half of a chocolate, eaten in this way, is as satisfying as two or three whole chocolates because the flavour (or taste) has been in your mouth for a long time.

After that sweet interlude let us look at lunch. Suppose that we have another traditional meal – fish and chips:

Plaice (battered), deep-fried	170 g (6 oz)	635 calories
Chips	140 g (5 oz)	435 calories
Total		1070 calories

A smaller portion:

Plaice (battered), deep-fried	115 g (4 oz)	425 calories
Chips	85 g (3 oz)	260 calories
Total		685 calories

Now if the fish is grilled instead of fried and if we use larger chips (which, because the total surface area is smaller, soak up less fat):

Plaice (battered), grilled	115 g (4 oz)	190 calories
Chips, large	85 g (3 oz)	115 calories
Total		305 calories

Thus we save 385 calories by eating a little less and a further 380 calories by cooking more sensibly, a total saving of 765 calories on *one* dish! If this is followed by coffee once again 95 calories can be saved, making a grand total saving of 860 calories.

Now, afternoon tea:

Cream doughnut	85 g (3 oz)	355 calories

If you do not eat all of it:

Cream doughnut	55 g (2 oz)	240 calories

A saving of 115 calories. With this you may drink a cup of tea:

Tea	140 g (5 oz)	5 calories
+ milk	30 g (1 oz)	20 calories
+ sugar	10 g (2 tspns)	60 calories
Total		85 calories

Using low-calorie substitutes:

Tea	140 g (5 oz)	5 calories
+ skimmed milk	30 g (1 oz)	10 calories
+ artificial sweetener		0 calories
Total		15 calories

A saving of 70 calories on the cup of tea, and a total saving for afternoon tea of 185 calories.

Now, supper:

Tomato soup (cream)	285 g (10 oz)	420 calories

A smaller portion:

Tomato soup (cream)	200 g (7 oz)	295 calories

Using a low-calorie substitute:

Low-calorie tomato soup	200 g (7 oz)	50 calories

Saving 125 calories by eating less and a further 245 calories by using a low-calorie brand. Followed by:

Hamburgers (medium size), fried	2	320 calories
Potatoes, mashed	140 g (5 oz)	170 calories
Mushrooms, fried	55 g (2 oz)	65 calories
Tomatoes, fried	115 g (4 oz)	80 calories
Total		635 calories

With smaller portions:

Hamburgers (medium size), fried	1½	240 calories
Potatoes, mashed	85 g (3 oz)	100 calories
Mushrooms, fried	45 g (1½ oz)	50 calories
Tomatoes, fried	85 g (3 oz)	60 calories
Total		**450 calories**

(At this point it is useful to illustrate a point made earlier – namely that some foods are less helpful than others when eaten less. Compare the effect of eating smaller portions of the above-mentioned vegetables with, say:

Cabbage	115 g (4 oz)	8 calories	55 g (2 oz)	4 calories
Carrots	85 g (3 oz)	18 calories	45 g (1½ oz)	9 calories
Lettuce	10 g (¼ oz)	1 calorie	5 g (⅛ oz)	½ calorie
Total		**27 calories**		**13½ calories**

A total saving of 13½ calories compared with 105 calories saved on the potatoes, mushrooms and tomatoes above.) To return to our original supper, if we grill instead of fry the food and if we have baked instead of mashed potato (giving us the added bonus of preserving more of its vitamin C content):

Hamburgers (medium size, frozen), grilled	1½	135 calories
Baked potato (without butter or cream)	85 g (3 oz)	70 calories
Mushrooms, grilled	45 g (1½ oz)	5 calories
Tomatoes, grilled	85 g (3 oz)	10 calories
Total		**220 calories**

Thus a saving of 185 calories by eating less, and a further 230 calories by cooking in a slightly different way – a total saving of 415 calories.

To follow, apple pie with cream:

Apple pie	140 g (5 oz)	270 calories
Cream	55 g (2 oz)	465 calories
Total		735 calories

Eating a little less:

Apple pie	85 g (3 oz)	160 calories
Cream	30 g (1 oz)	230 calories
Total		390 calories

A saving of 345 calories. Followed by coffee, with its saving of 95 calories, a total of 1225 calories can be saved in this four-course supper.

Of course alcoholic drinks are another area in which calorie savings can be made. In Chapter 17 you will find calorie values of common alcoholic drinks. Once again, you can save calories by either drinking less or substituting low-calorie drinks. For example, using a low-calorie tonic water in your gin and tonic can save you about 60 calories. Similarly, one pint of light ale in preference to strong ale can save over 250 calories. With regard to beer it should be remembered that diabetic beers and lagers are high in calorific content because they are made by fermenting the carbohydrate that is present in beer (as distinct from the alcohol) into alcohol. Because carbohydrates yield only four calories per gram (compared with alcohol's seven calories per gram) the total calorie content is thus increased.

Once again it must be stressed that there is no need for you to count calories in the way that has been done here. The calories have been counted in some typical meals merely to illustrate the principles of eating less. Again, it must be emphasized that you can continue to eat all your favourite foods. Simply eat a little less of them. Incidentally some foods contain negligible calories and you do not have to worry about eating less of them (these are listed at the end of Chapter 17).

The first edition of this book virtually ended at this point. All that followed was a number of psychological aids or 'tricks' which were helpful in cutting down food intake painlessly. The book, though profoundly simple, was looked upon as something of a revelation because no one had previously written a 'no diet' slimming book. The book appealed to many people who found that it helped them to lose weight painlessly and permanently.

But, since that first edition, I have found that some slimmers need more detailed advice about the psychological aspects of slimming. I have gradually devised a series of eating 'hints' which almost every slimmer will find useful, and these form Chapter 15 of this book.

Another useful addition in this book is one week's menus (Chapter 16). These illustrate further some of the calorie-saving principles described in this chapter and they also demonstrate that your food can be both economical (in terms of calories) *and* delicious.

Chapters 14, 15 and 16 are the heart of my approach to slimming. Read them carefully and follow the advice contained in them. The result? Very soon you will be eating all the foods that you enjoy eating. You will not be counting calories. You will be eating healthily. You will be eating (and drinking) happily.

And you will be losing weight – without really dieting.

15

Eating hints

The only useful stimulus, or cue, to eating is hunger. The problem is that we have conditioned ourselves to respond to other cues also. These cues, which include habit, social custom, boredom, anger, and so on, are irrelevant and inappropriate as regards our bodies' food requirements. In addition, we have lost the ability to recognize and respond to the disappearance of hunger which should be the cue to stop eating. Animals which live in the wild never become overweight. A lion, for example, will go without food for two or three days. Only when it is hungry will it hunt and kill to provide a meal. And it will stop eating once it is no longer hungry even if there is some meat still left on the carcass. The lion is using hunger as its control for when to start and when to stop eating. Similarly a breast-fed baby will suck only when he or she is hungry and stops sucking when that hunger is satisfied.

In this chapter we will examine many of the cues relating to eating that we encounter every day. Some are good, but most are bad. We need to encourage the good ones and to suppress the bad ones. In order to do this effectively, let us look at each cue in turn and see what we should do either to encourage or to suppress it.

It is perhaps best to consider the cues in some kind of chronological order. So we shall start with the actual purchase of food, moving on to the planning of mealtimes, then the consumption of the food, and finally to the disposal of what is left. It is useful to consider the cues in terms of what you can do about them, that is, how you can eliminate or suppress the undesirable ones and how you can encourage the useful ones. These ways of modifying eating behaviour I shall describe as 'hints'.

First let us think about behaviour when buying food. It is an interesting fact that people who shop after a meal, when they are not hungry, buy less food.

Hint 1: Shop for food as soon as possible after a meal rather than when your stomach is empty

The human mind is easily persuaded by colourful and attractive foods to buy foods which were not originally intended to be bought.

Hint 2: Make a list of the foods you intend to buy. Keep that list in your hand whilst shopping and stick rigidly to it

Hint 3: Limit the amount of money you take with you to that which you will need for the food on your list and no more

I once had a patient who, when she was out, could never walk past a shop that sold food without going in and buying some. I told her that if she was not out for the specific purpose of buying food she should leave her purse at home. It is a good idea to decide in advance which shops you will go into to buy your food and name these shops on your list.

Hint 4: List the shops at which you intend to buy food and do not enter other food shops

Planning your meals each day is very important. It is not so much *what* you eat at these meals but *when* you eat. The idea is to satisfy your hunger at proper meals and so avoid between-meal snacks. Also, skipped meals cause excessive hunger, which in turn leads to gorging. Very often the person who only has a cup of coffee for breakfast, and no lunch, will be so hungry by the evening that more food will be eaten at the evening meal than might otherwise have been eaten in three meals (when the total calorie intake might well have been less than that in one meal a day).

Hint 5: Avoid excessive hunger by having regular, planned meals. Plan these meals daily and stick to them

Central to the whole concept of modifying eating behaviour is the idea that you eat only if you are hungry. It is amazing how much food many of us eat when we are not in fact hungry. And this food represents the calories that are largely responsible for excess weight.

Hint 6: Eat only if and when you are hungry. If you are not hungry, do not eat

In fact, with say three planned meals a day, each of which need only be fairly light, you are almost certain to feel at least a little hungry at mealtimes. But once you embark on a meal the use of hunger as your control does not end. You have to stop eating when you are no longer hungry, an important point we shall examine in more detail shortly (Hint 13).

It is very tempting to 'overdraw' on your calories in advance, so that perhaps you justify a mid-morning snack by saying to yourself that it can be instead of your lunchtime pudding. The chances are than when it comes to lunch you will still have your pudding. If you wish, forget your pudding at lunchtime so that you can allow yourself a teatime snack, although personally I think that the practice of having snacks at all is dangerous for someone trying to control his weight. You need very firm self-control to indulge safely in this habit.

Hint 7: Do not overdraw on your calories in advance

Let us look now at the actual food that you eat. At this point I am not going to go into detail about ways of preparing food that save calories because such matters are covered fully in other chapters. I merely want to draw your attention to one point concerning low-calorie foods which is useful to remember each day and should be considered as another Hint.

Low-calorie foods can be boring. They can also be made very attractive and interesting if they are 'dressed up' with imaginative low-calorie garnishes such as parsley or paprika. You can really let your imagination run riot here!

Hint 8: Make low-calorie foods more interesting by using imaginative low-calorie garnishes

Let us look now at eating behaviour during meals. This is the most important area of all because there are many opportunities for modifying your eating behaviour.

The first important point to consider is *where* you actually eat. It is vital that you look upon eating as an 'activity', with its time and *place*, as you would any other activity. For example, you play squash on a squash court. You swim in a swimming pool. You drive a car on a road. You sleep in your bedroom. You wash in the bathroom. You go to the lavatory in the small room built for that sole purpose. So, in the same way, you eat in your 'eating room' which is *one* room and one room only, probably either the dining-room *or* the breakfast room *or* the kitchen. Do not vary. Whenever you eat at home always eat in the same room every time.

Hint 9: When eating at home, eat all your meals in one room in the house only

The idea of eating in one room only carries greater force if you extend it further so that you always eat while sitting on the same chair at the same position at the table. This space in your home becomes your personal 'eating area'.

Hint 10: Always eat in the same place in the one room in which you have your meals

The next two hints help reinforce Hint 10 because they emphasize that you can eat only while *sitting* at a table

Hint 11: Eat only when you are sitting at a dining-table.
Hint 12: Never put anything in your mouth (except a tooth-brush) while you are standing

As I said earlier in this chapter, central to the whole concept of modifying eating behaviour is the idea that you eat only when you are hungry (see Hint 6). But, of course, deciding whether or not you are hungry is not just a once-and-for-all decision taken before you start a meal. Just as hunger is the cue to eat, so the lack of hunger, or its disappearance or satisfaction, should be the cue to stop eating. But you can only decide that you are no longer hungry, and therefore that you should stop eating, if, during the course of the meal, you repeatedly ask yourself the question, 'Am I still hungry?' The moment that your honest answer is no is the moment that you should stop eating. Thus:

> Hint 13: While eating, periodically ask yourself, 'Am I still hungry?' If your honest answer is no, stop eating

Of all the hints, Hint 13 is the single most important. The lack of its observance is probably the main reason that most people become overweight. And it is equally probable that it is the main reason that so many people have difficulty in losing weight. Its importance cannot be stressed too much and I would strongly urge you to devote as much time to thinking about Hint 13 as the time for all the other hints put together.

One of the main reasons that people have difficulty with Hint 13 is that it goes against the grain to leave food on the plate. We have been brought up to regard it as wrong, unwholesome or just plain ill-mannered to leave food on the plate. Our parents thought there was something wrong with us if we did so. Hosts worry that perhaps you do not enjoy their cooking. Or, if in a restaurant, it is simply a waste of money to leave all that delicious food. Business lunches appear to be a particularly difficult problem. People worry that their colleagues or clients will think them either discourteous or in poor health.

One of my patients admitted to me that one of his main hazards was eating out in friends' homes. He was always far too polite ever to refuse anything. In fact, he was a popular guest who was never short of dinner invitations because his hosts knew that he would always eat everything, which they found very flattering. Doting relatives often present difficult challenges to slimmers. A good appetite, they feel, is a sign of good health and, if food is refused, galloping paranoia sets in and they assume that there must be something wrong with their cooking. And yet members of the Royal Family, who probably have more social dining at huge banquets than almost anyone else, and who at all times exercise the utmost tact and diplomacy, follow Hint 13 absolutely strictly. Only two or three mouthfuls are eaten of each of the five or six courses, the rest of the food being left on the plates. Thus the meal is 'paced' so that enough hunger is left for each succeeding course. In this way *every* course, even pudding, can be tasted and enjoyed. A variant of this hint is used by a world-famous American singer. He takes a knife and draws a line down the middle of every plateful of solid food that he is given. Half the food he eats, and the other half is returned to the kitchen from whence it came.

In order to be able to apply Hint 13, clearly you must remain fully aware at all times during a meal of your degree of hunger. Your mind must be concentrated, your thoughts focused on this matter. This can be achieved only if your attention is totally undivided, only if one hundred per cent of your consciousness is devoted to the question of whether or not you are hungry. Reading at the table, watching television, solving a crossword puzzle are activities which demand your attention and potentially undermine your ability to focus on your hunger. Chatting of course is allowed but try to avoid discussion of a serious nature.

Hint 14: Allow no other activity to take place while you are
eating

Observance of Hint 14 will also help to heighten your enjoyment of food.

Another important aid to concentrating the mind and ensuring that food is never eaten mindlessly, and therefore when you are possibly not even hungry, is to ensure that you always eat solid food with a knife, fork or spoon. *Never* use your fingers. Using utensils makes you think much more about the fact that you are eating, whereas putting food into your mouth with your fingers does not psychologically seem so much like eating. It is amazing how many peanuts will disappear from a bowl down your throat without you noticing. Observance of this principle should extend even to the eating of a sandwich which, ridiculous as it may seem, should be eaten with a knife and fork. Making it an open sandwich makes it appear less ridiculous!

Hint 15: Always use a knife, fork or spoon for *all* solid food

Time-limiting and delaying strategies are very useful aids in limiting food intake. An obvious one is to impose a limit of, say, ten minutes for breakfast, twenty minutes for lunch, and again twenty minutes for supper or dinner (ensuring of course that you do not gobble to take in more food!):

Hint 16: Limit the time you allow yourself for each meal

A further delaying strategy is to make the actual acquisition of food at mealtimes difficult for yourself. For example, at breakfast, toast only one slice of bread (or even only half a slice) at a time. When you have eaten that then go back to the toaster and put in another slice of bread and wait by the toaster until the toast is ready. In this way you will not want the bother of eating several slices of toast, whereas you would have been more likely to eat more had you made several slices of toast simultaneously. One of my patients keeps her toaster upstairs. Every time she wants another slice of toast she has to go upstairs to make it and she brings it downstairs to eat it!

Hint 17: Make the acquisition of food at mealtimes difficult for yourself

The more quickly food is eaten, the greater the amount that is eaten. People who never put down their knives and forks, but who busy themselves by cutting up and preparing their next mouthful while still chewing, tend to eat food quickly and therefore eat more of it. It is a good delaying strategy to put down your knife and fork between mouthfuls for a period of, say, one or two minutes.

Hint 18: Put down your knife, fork or spoon for a prescribed period between mouthfuls

Another delaying tactic is to cut your food up into many small pieces. This has the effect of making your plate look as if there is more food on it than there actually is, and the process of cutting up food takes time, leaving you with less time to actually eat in.

Hint 19: Cut up your food into as many small pieces as you
can

Another useful strategy for making your plate look as if there is more food on it than is actually there is to use a small plate and spread your food evenly over the plate.

Hint 20: Serve your food on to a small plate and spread the
food evenly over the plate

When serving yourself it is a good idea to use small, measured quantities – say, one or two tablespoons of mashed potato, for example – rather than helping yourself *ad lib* from a large serving bowl.

Hint 21: Serve yourself small, measured quantities of food
rather than helping yourself *ad lib*

Remove the temptation to help yourself to further helpings of food after you have begun eating.

Hint 22: Do not keep serving dishes on the table while you
eat

Returning to delaying tactics, it is said that Gladstone used an excellent one, which was to chew each mouthful until it turned to water!

Hint 23: Chew each mouthful for as long as possible

And talking of mouthfuls, it is a good idea to count how many mouthfuls you eat in, say, two, three or five minutes and then to try to reduce that number, so that you eat more slowly.

Hint 24: Count how many mouthfuls you eat in a prescribed
period. Reduce the number of mouthfuls, so that
you eat more slowly

Delaying strategies centred around mouthfuls can reach almost Freudian proportions, but there is one more which deserves consideration. This is to make a point of swallowing all the food in your mouth before you put any more food into it.

Hint 25: Ensure that all the food from each mouthful is swallowed before you put any more food into your mouth

One patient told me of a revealing way of discovering how quickly she ate her food. She placed her table under a wall-mounted mirror and watched herself eating. She was appalled by the sight of herself gobbling her food, scarcely pausing to breathe between mouthfuls, and seemingly shovelling her food into her mouth. I have since recommended the 'mirror ploy' to some of my other patients all of whom have found the experience equally revealing and salutary!

Even after you have decided that you are no longer hungry it is very tempting to pick at food so long as it remains in front of you. This applies to children's leftovers too: mothers are notorious for picking at these!

Hint 26: After finishing your meal dispose of any leftovers immediately

An extension of this principle provides the next hint:

Hint 27: Leave the table as soon as you have finished eating. If you can, leave the table between courses

Returning to children, if they ask you for any chocolates, sweets, nuts, and so on, tell them to get them for themselves (assuming, of course, that they are old enough to do so). You must try to avoid putting yourself into direct contact with foods which may tempt you.

Hint 28: Let *others*, especially children (if old enough), get their own chocolates, sweets and nuts from the cupboard

If you feel tempted to have chocolates yourself, and you feel that your conscience will allow this, then at least limit the number you have. Don't leave an open box of chocolates in front of you: it is surprising how easily the chocolates will disappear into your mouth before you even realize it. Take the chocolate (or chocolates) that you are going to eat out of the box and then *put the box away out of sight* before you start to eat any of them. Savour each chocolate (which, after all, you are eating only for its taste). Nibble the chocolate, bit by bit, roll it around your mouth with your tongue, and try not to let your mind be distracted away from the business of eating and enjoying it. In this way you will obtain maximum pleasure from perhaps only one chocolate and there will be no need for you to plough your way through a boxful.

If you think that eating a chocolate is something that only occurs to you when you see a box of chocolates, or if you know that you have a box in the cupboard, *don't keep chocolates (or sweets) in the home at all*! What isn't there can't be eaten! In fact, it is not a bad idea to try to avoid all 'snackable' foods in the home, keeping only those foods which take time to prepare.

Many of the purely eating hints I have described are delaying tactics, and these are central to modifying eating behaviour. There are two reasons why this is so. First, they ensure that you eat less food. Second, and equally important, they actually help increase your enjoyment of food. An excuse I often hear from people who fail to lose weight is, 'I enjoy my food too much.' If that has a familiar ring, stop for a moment to consider the difference between a *gourmet* and a *gourmand*. A gourmand is a glutton who eats anything and everything. A gourmet, on the other hand, is a connoisseur and is highly selective about food, enjoyment coming not from the quantity of food, but its flavour, smell, texture, and appearance. A gourmet in fact eats *less* food than a gourmand but enjoys it more. Next time you eat in a restaurant have a look at how other people eat. The fast indiscriminate eaters who eat more mouthfuls in any given time and chew each mouthful less than others are generally the fat ones, whereas the slow thoughtful eaters are usually the slim ones. You do not need quantity, but quality, to enjoy your food. As Sir Walter A. Raleigh (not the Elizabethan but the late nineteenth- and early twentieth-century writer) wrote in *Laughter from a Cloud*:

Eat slowly: only men in rags
And gluttons old in sin
Mistake themselves for carpet bags
And tumble victuals in.

Don't allow yourself to be a carpet bag!

Unfortunately no amount of hints or ploys seem to be enough for some slimmers who find their resolve weakening from time to time. If you find yourself belonging to this small minority you may find the following ploy helpful! *A nylon cord*. This can be useful when you have already lost weight and then find yourself starting to regain weight. It owes its origin to slim photographic models, some of whom tie a thin gold chain around their waists. If the chain becomes tighter, they know that they are putting on weight. Fortunately a nylon cord works just as well without burning a hole in your pocket! Tie the nylon cord around your waist. The cord should be fairly thin (about 2 mm) so that it does not show through your clothes. (Such a cord is easily obtained in a haberdashery shop.) Tie it sufficiently tightly that when you are sitting it causes a white (but not red) line to be visible in your skin. When you lie down it should cause no indentation. Keep the cord on at all times, even when you have a bath. Every few days, as you lose weight, tighten it a little more. If, while you are still trying to lose weight or after you have reached your target weight, the cord becomes tighter, you will know that your weight is starting to creep up again. Do not forget, if you are a woman, that as a result of fluid retention there may be some increase in your waist premenstrually, and make allowance for this.

And now we come to the last of the hints. As I have said several times in this book, boredom is the chief enemy of the slimmer. Eating just for something to do, the dreaded snacking impulse, is born of boredom. If boredom is a regular feature of your life it is worth spending some time examining your lifestyle. Do you, for example, at the end of the day, slump in a chair with a box of chocolates by your side as you watch television? Do you automatically head for the fridge and look for 'goodies'? If so, try to think up alternative activities. Why not go out and cut the grass, water the plants, write a letter, or go out on an evening course? Do some chore such as clearing out the garage, or read a book, or have a bath. Go for a walk. Notice the scenery and observe so many details that in the normal hustle and bustle of daily life you miss. Take up tennis, or bowling, or cycling.

Try to adopt a really positive attitude towards your lifestyle, so that healthy, calorie-burning activities are substituted for unhealthy, calorie-consuming ones. The result will be a fitter, slimmer you who will probably enjoy life all the more.

Hint 29: Adopt a positive attitude. Exchange calorie-burning activities for calorie-consuming ones. Modify your whole lifestyle to this end, and enjoy your life all the more

16

Menus and recipes illustrating the dietary principles of How to lose weight without really dieting

On the following pages are some menu and recipe ideas. It is not intended that they should necessarily be followed, since my approach to slimming is that you eat more or less what you like, only a little less of it. The purpose of the menus and recipes is to show how you can save calories whilst at the same time enjoying *normal*, as opposed to 'diet', food. Calorie counts are given simply to illustrate the calorie savings.

Some of you may actually wish to follow these menus. I use an approximate 1250 calories a day (give or take about 100 calories) as the basis, and I will show how you may increase your intake to about 1500 calories or decrease it to about 1000 calories.

Current medical opinion is that meat should be limited to four times a week, and this is reflected in the week's menus. But for those of you who simply cannot live without meat every day I have given meat alternatives to the two vegetarian main dishes.

The menus demonstrate how delicious and varied your choice of dishes can be. In particular you will notice that:

there is no need to depend on salads
there is no need to cut out potatoes

Although alcohol is not specifically mentioned there is no need to cut it out. However you must remember that alcohol is calorific, and I would suggest that if you would like wine with your main meal substitute 2–3 glasses for the bread roll in the following examples.

A useful tip: a small bowl of chopped up raw vegetables (for example, carrots, red or green peppers, gherkins, celery) at the table is a useful low-calorie filler to accompany your lunchtime snack. Chewing a couple of sticks of celery will use up almost as many calories as they contain!

If you think in terms of moderation, you can see how easy it is to lose weight and enjoy your food.

The figure after each dish is the calorie value of that dish.

Sunday

Breakfast

Shredded wheat (p. 138)	110
Toast and honey	100
Coffee or tea with skimmed milk	20

Lunch

Roast beef	300
Roast potatoes (115 g, 4 oz)	180
Peas (115 g, 4 oz)	50
Yorkshire pudding (p. 153)	110
Apple and lemon compote (p. 163)	50

Supper

Cheese on toast (p. 144)	200
1 (wholemeal) bread roll	215

Total	1335

On 1000 calories a day, skip the roll. On 1500 calories, allow yourself guacamole with crudités (p. 149) as your first course at lunch.

Monday

Breakfast

Home-made muesli (p. 139)	130
Toast and marmalade (p. 140)	100
Coffee or tea with skimmed milk*	20

* All these sample menus assume coffee or tea *without* sugar but with optional artificial sweetener

Lunch

Orange juice (225 ml, 8 oz)	85
Jacket potato with Edam cheese & apple and cabbage slaw (p. 142)	175
Coffee with skimmed milk	20

Supper

Minestrone (p. 148)	180
Beef & wine casserole (p. 152)	265
Peach melba (p. 159)	100
1 (wholemeal) bread roll	215

Total	1290

On 1000 calories a day, skip the roll. On 1500 calories, allow yourself a wholemeal bread roll (215 calories) at lunch.

Tuesday

Breakfast

Shredded wheat (p. 138)	120
Tea with skimmed milk	20

Lunch

Apricot salad (p. 147)	65
2 slices wholemeal bread with low-fat spread	180
Coffee with skimmed milk	20

Supper

Smoked mackerel pâté (p. 150)	140
2 slices wholemeal toast	120
Mushroom and onion bake (p. 158)	250
1 jacket potato	250
Fruit salad (p. 160)	75

Total	1240

Alternative to Mushroom and onion bake and jacket potato:

Veal in breadcrumbs (p. 153)	255
Mashed potatoes (115 g, 4 oz)	135
Boiled parsnips (115 g, 4 oz)	65
Sweetcorn (55 g, 2 oz)	65

Have just *one* slice of toast with the pâté. Daily total: 1200 calories.

On 1000 calories a day, have just *one* slice of bread with lunch and *one* slice of toast with supper. On 1500 calories, allow yourself additional toast and Gentleman's Relish (90 calories, p. 140) for breakfast and a glass of fruit juice (85 calories) with your supper.

Wednesday

Breakfast

Melon and orange waker (p. 141)	110
Kedgeree (p. 141)	180
Coffee or tea with skimmed milk	20

Lunch

Pasta and chicken salad (p. 147)	235
Coffee with skimmed milk	20

Supper

French onion soup (p. 150)	50
Roast lamb with garlic (p. 154)	300
Broccoli (115 g, 4 oz)	20
Peas (115 g, 4 oz)	50
Lemon jelly with banana (p. 160)	30
1 (wholemeal) bread roll	215

	Total	1230

On 1000 calories a day, skip the roll. On 1500 calories, allow yourself a wholemeal bread roll (215 calories) at lunch.

Thursday

Breakfast

Weetabix (with or without bran) (p. 138)	80
Kipper and lemon (p. 141)	90
Coffee or tea with skimmed milk	20

Lunch

Chicken and apple and cabbage slaw sandwich (p. 142)	280
Coffee with skimmed milk	20

Supper

Grapefruit cocktail (p. 151)	60
Vegetable lasagne (p. 157)	455
Green salad	15
Fruit Pavlova (p. 160)	115
1 (wholemeal) bread roll	215

	Total	1350

Alternative to Lasagne and salad:

Spaghetti Bolognese (p. 155)	430

Daily total: 1310 calories.

Incidentally, if preferred you can use the lasagne sauce on the spaghetti instead of bolognese sauce.

On 1000 calories a day, skip the roll. On 1500 calories, allow yourself a fruit juice starter (85 calories) for lunch.

Friday

Breakfast

Instant porridge (with or without bran) (p. 139)	165
Coffee or tea with skimmed milk	20

Lunch

Orange juice (225 ml, 8 oz)	85
Cottage cheese, radish and cucumber sandwich (p. 142)	240
Coffee with skimmed milk	20

Supper

Leeks à la Grecque (p. 151)	60
Lemon chicken (p. 156)	210
Boiled potatoes (115 g, 4 oz)	90
Peas (115 g, 4 oz)	50
Chocolate soufflé (p. 161)	90
1 (wholemeal) bread roll	215

	Total	1245

On 1000 calories a day, skip the roll. On 1500 calories, allow yourself toast and marmalade (100 calories) for breakfast and an additional vegetable at supper.

Saturday

Breakfast

Home-made muesli (p. 139)	130
Sausage and tomato (p. 140)	165
Coffee or tea with skimmed milk	20

Lunch

Jacket potato with bacon (p. 144)	300
Coffee with skimmed milk	20

Supper

Fillet of sole with mushrooms (p. 157)	145
New potatoes (115 g, 4 oz)	90
Mixed salad	20
2 Crêpes Suzettes (p. 162)	140
1 (wholemeal) bread roll	215

	Total	1245

On 1000 calories a day, skip the roll. On 1500 calories, allow yourself cream of mushroom soup (190 calories, p. 148) as a supper starter.

BREAKFASTS

Breakfast is the most important meal as it marks the start of a new day. Do not be tempted to skip it. Besides, by using skimmed milk, artificial sweeteners, low-fat spreads, and grilling instead of frying, you can keep the calorie, saturated fat and cholesterol intake down quite easily. So it really is not worth trying to get through the morning with an unpleasantly empty stomach. (Incidentally, powdered or granulated artificial sweeteners are more convenient than liquid forms for use on cereals.)

The method of putting the ingredients together in some of the recipes that follow may seem too obvious to state. The reason, however, for describing how to prepare cereal or toast or a sandwich is to demonstrate the use of small quantities and low-calorie substitutes in order to save calories.

Weetabix (and bran)

1 Weetabix
(15 g (½ oz) bran)
55 ml (2 oz) skimmed milk
granulated artificial sweetener

Sprinkle the sweetener to taste over the Weetabix and serve with hot or cold skimmed milk. Optional bran may be sprinkled over the Weetabix.

Serves 1: 80 calories

Shredded wheat (with bran)

1 shredded wheat
(15 g (½ oz) bran)
55 ml (2 oz) skimmed milk
granulated artificial sweetener

Serve as in the previous breakfast.

Serves 1: 110 calories

Instant porridge (with bran)

30 g (1 oz) Ready Brek
(15 g (½ oz) bran)
140 ml (¼ pint) skimmed milk
granulated artificial sweetener

Serve as in the previous breakfast.

Serves 1: 165 calories

Muesli

30 g (1 oz) muesli
55 ml (2 oz) skimmed milk
granulated artificial sweetener

Sprinkle the sweetener to taste over the muesli and serve
with hot or cold skimmed milk.

Serves 1: 130 calories

Home-made muesli

55 g (2 oz) porridge oats
285 ml (½ pint) unsweetened orange juice or apple juice
55 g (2 oz) dried fruit, e.g. sultanas
30 g (1 oz) nuts, e.g. hazelnuts
2 apples (chopped but not peeled) or 1 small banana
140 ml (¼ pint) skimmed milk

Pour the juice over the oats and leave overnight. In the
morning stir in the dried fruit, crushed nuts and chopped
apple or banana. Divide into four portions and serve with
one-quarter of the milk on each portion. No added sweetener
should be necessary as the fruit will provide a lot of natural
sweetness.

Serves 4: 130 calories per portion

Toast and marmalade

1 slice of wholemeal bread
7·5 g (¼ oz) low-fat margarine
5 g (1 *level* tspn) marmalade

Toast the bread and spread with margarine and marmalade.

Serves 1: 100 calories

Toast and Gentleman's Relish

1 slice of wholemeal bread
7·5 g (¼ oz) low-fat margarine
Gentleman's Relish to taste

Toast the bread and spread with margarine and Gentleman's Relish.

Serves 1: 90 calories

Toast and honey

1 slice of wholemeal bread
7·5 g (¼ oz) low-fat margarine
5 g (1 *level* tspn) honey

Toast the bread and spread with margarine and honey.

Serves 1: 100 calories

Sausage and tomato

2 chipolatas
1 tomato
basil

Prick the sausages and grill. When they are almost cooked halve the tomato, sprinkle with basil, and place on the grill pan beside the sausages. Cook for about 5 minutes. Serve the sausages and tomato together.

Serves 1: 165 calories

Anyone not very familiar with grilling food will be amazed at the amount of fat (and therefore calories too) that is lost. A normal portion of fried bacon, for example, would give you nearly 100 extra calories compared with grilled bacon. There really is no reason to fry foods such as bacon, sausages, burgers, and so on, as they all taste better and are healthier for you if grilled.

Kipper and lemon

1 small kipper
½ lemon

Grill the kipper until cooked and serve with slices of lemon.

Serves 1: 90 calories

Kedgeree

225 g (8 oz) smoked haddock
115 g (4 oz) cooked rice
salt
freshly milled black pepper
1 slice lemon

Cook the fish, then skin and flake it. Mix the fish with the rice, and season it with salt and pepper. Garnish the kedgeree with a slice of lemon.

Serves 2: 180 calories per portion

Melon and orange waker
(A good one for warm sunny mornings!)

1 small melon
1 orange
4 slices wholemeal bread (or rolls)
30 g (1 oz) low-fat margarine

Slice the melon and cut into cubes. Peel the orange and cut into slices. Place the melon cubes in 4 glass bowls and decorate with the orange slices. Serve with a slice of wholemeal bread or roll. Substitute an apple or small banana for the orange if you prefer.

Serves 4: 110 calories per portion

Sandwiches and snacks

First, a brief word on what I mean by 'snacks'. These are *not* things to eat between meals but are the meals themselves. A snack simply denotes a meal which, though nutritious and satisfying, is fairly modest in size. Moreover it can be prepared quickly and easily. And yet, although it can be almost literally 'thrown together' it offers great scope for culinary imagination.

Sandwiches

Sandwiches can be varied and nutritious providing the fillings are sensibly thought out. Try to use wholemeal bread and low-fat spreads.

The basic method for making each sandwich described is as follows:

Ingredients
2 slices wholemeal bread
15 g (½ oz) low-fat margarine
filling

Method
Spread the bread with the margarine. Place the filling on one slice of bread and then put the remaining slice on top. Cut into four and serve.

Chicken and apple and cabbage slaw sandwich

2 slices cooked chicken
30 g (1 oz) apple and cabbage slaw (see below)

Serves 1: 90 calories

Apple and cabbage slaw

1 small white cabbage
3 red apples
15 ml (1 tbspn) lemon juice
40 ml (3 tbspns) low-calorie mayonnaise (p. 163)
40 ml (3 tbspns) natural low-fat yoghurt

Shred the cabbage finely and put it into a bowl. Core the apples and slice them thinly. Dip them in the lemon juice to prevent browning and add them to the cabbage. Mix the low-calorie mayonnaise with the yoghurt and gently stir into the apple and cabbage mixture.

Serves 4: 65 calories per portion

Low-fat cheese, radish and cucumber sandwich

55 g (2 oz) low-fat cheese, e.g. cottage cheese
4 radishes
4 slices cucumber

Serves 1: 240 calories

Hot snacks

Hot snacks based on jacket potatoes really are quick, easy and very delicious as well as being good for you. Don't listen to the old-fashioned nonsense about the need to cut out potatoes from your diet if you want to lose weight. A medium-sized potato baked in the oven until it is soft to the touch and then served in either of the following ways is very nutritious without being particularly calorific. But don't forget to eat the skin – it is a very useful source of fibre.

Jacket potato with Edam cheese and apple and cabbage slaw

1 medium potato
15 g (½ oz) low-fat margarine
30 g (1 oz) Edam cheese
30 g (1 oz) apple and cabbage slaw

Cook the potato in the oven, gas mark 6, 400°F (200°C), for 45 to 60 minutes until soft to the touch. Slice the potato in half, mash in a little margarine and serve with grated cheese sprinkled on top with apple and cabbage slaw. If you use home-made apple and cabbage slaw, dress with a low-calorie dressing. If you use a commercial coleslaw choose one with vinaigrette or a low-calorie dressing (p. 163).

Serves 1: 175 calories

143

Jacket potato and bacon

1 medium potato
15 g (½ oz) low-fat margarine
2 rashers lean back bacon

Cook the potato in the oven, gas mark 6, 400°F (200°C), for 45 to 60 minutes until soft to the touch. Slice the potato in half, mash in a little margarine and serve with crispy grilled bacon.

Serves 1: 300 calories

Mushrooms and tomato on toast

4 medium-sized mushrooms
4 tomatoes
30 g (1 oz) polyunsaturated margarine
freshly milled black pepper
4 slices wholemeal bread

Slice the mushrooms and tomato and fry them gently in the margarine for about 5 minutes. Season and serve on toasted bread.

Serves 4: 90 calories per portion

Cheese on toast

15 g (½ oz) polyunsaturated margarine
15 g (½ oz) flour
45 ml (3 tbspns) skimmed milk
115 g (4 oz) low-fat cheese, e.g. cottage cheese
5 g (1 tspn) mustard
Worcestershire sauce
salt
freshly milled black pepper
2 slices wholemeal bread

Melt the margarine in a saucepan, add the flour and stir in the milk. Cook gently for two minutes, then beat in the cheese and season to taste. To serve pour over the toasted bread.

Serves 2: 200 calories

Salads as main courses or snacks

When preparing the ingredients for salads always leave the skins on the fruit and vegetables, wherever possible, as they provide useful roughage.

Carrot salad

4 large carrots
55 g (2 oz) seedless raisins
30 g (1 tbspn) chopped parsley
15 ml (½ tbspn) lemon juice
salt
pepper

Peel and grate the carrots. Put the carrots into a bowl, add the raisins and parsley, sprinkle on the lemon juice, and give the ingredients a good stir.

Serves 4: 40 calories per portion

Red pepper and beanshoot salad

1 red pepper
225 g (8 oz) beanshoots
30 ml (2 tbspns) home-made low-calorie vinaigrette dressing (see p. 163)

Finely slice the pepper and put it into a bowl with the beanshoots. Add the vinaigrette dressing and toss well.

Serves 4: 20 calories per portion

Tomato salad

455 g (1 lb) ripe tomatoes
1 large onion
15 g (1 tbspn) chopped parsley
30 ml (2 tbspns) lemon juice
salt
freshly milled black pepper

Slice the tomatoes and place in four bowls. Slice the onion into rings and place on top of the tomatoes. Just before serving, sprinkle with lemon juice, parsley, salt and pepper.

Serves 4: 20 calories per portion

Celery, radish and green pepper salad

4 sticks celery
12 radishes
1 green pepper
15 ml (1 tbspn) home-made low-calorie vinaigrette dressing (see p. 163) or lemon juice

Slice the celery into small even pieces, and slice the radishes and green pepper. Mix together in a bowl and add vinaigrette or lemon juice.

Serves 4: 5–10 calories per portion

Green salad

30 ml (2 tbspns) home-made low-calorie vinaigrette dressing (see p. 163)
1 clove garlic (crushed)
salt and pepper
15 g (1 tbspn) chopped parsley
1 lettuce
4 spring onions
1 bunch watercress

Make up the vinaigrette dressing, add the crushed garlic, seasoning and parsley, and allow to stand for about an hour. In a salad bowl, mix together the lettuce, spring onions and watercress. Pour over the dressing and turn the salad gently so that it all becomes evenly coated.

Serves 4: 15 calories per portion

Apricot salad

8 fresh apricots
225 g (8 oz) low-fat cheese, e.g. cottage cheese
½ lettuce

Chop the apricots and mix into the cottage cheese. Arrange
two or three lettuce leaves on four plates and divide the
cheese mixture into four. Put a portion on to the lettuce on
each plate.

When apricots are not available, substitute tinned
pineapple canned in its own juice (*not* syrup), or chopped
apple or even a little chopped melon. The addition of fruit
turns cottage cheese into a much more enjoyable
experience.

Serves 4: 65 calories per portion

Pasta and chicken salad

115 g (4 oz) wholewheat pasta rings or shells
225 g (8 oz) cooked chicken
2 red apples
2 sticks celery
salt
freshly milled black pepper
30 ml (2 tbspns) low-cholesterol mayonnaise (see p. 163)
15 ml (1 tbspn) natural low-fat yoghurt

Cook the pasta according to the instructions on the packet.
Leave to cool. Remove the skin from the chicken and cut the
flesh into bite-sized pieces. Core and dice the apple. Chop
the celery and mix with the pasta, chicken and apple. Season.
Add the mayonnaise mixed with yoghurt and evenly coat the
chicken-pasta mixture. Serve on a bed of lettuce.

Serves 4: 235 calories per portion

STARTERS

Cream of mushroom soup

1 small onion
225 g (8 oz) mushrooms
55 g (2 oz) flour
55 g (2 oz) polyunsaturated margarine
570 ml (1 pint) chicken stock
570 ml (1 pint) skimmed milk
salt and pepper
(The calorie count assumes that you use stock cubes.
However you may prefer to make your own real stock, and
clearly the calories will depend on how fat the meat is and
what vegetables you use. Alternatively vegetable bouillon
cubes and granules, free of added salt, flavourings and
preservatives, may be used: these are available from health
food shops.)

Skin and finely chop onion. Chop mushrooms. Melt margarine
in a saucepan and fry onion until soft. Add chopped
mushrooms and fry for 5 minutes. Add flour and stir well.
Slowly add stock and milk to the mixture, stirring all the time.
Add salt and pepper. Bring to the boil and simmer for 5
minutes.

Serves 4: 190 calories per portion

Minestrone soup

2 sticks celery
1 large carrot
1 medium-sized potato
1 onion
1 leek
¼ small cabbage
30 g (1 oz) polyunsaturated margarine
1 clove garlic (crushed)
salt and pepper
15 g (1 level tbspn) tomato purée

1 small tin of tomatoes
1 pinch dried herbs (mixed or basil)
1700 ml (3 pints) beef stock
1 small tin cannellini beans
115 g (4 oz) pasta (preferably wholewheat), pasta shapes,
broken spaghetti, macaroni, etc.
55 g (2 oz) Edam cheese

(The vegetable ingredients can be varied to suit your taste.
For example, if you loathe leeks but love celery, leave out the
leek and add an extra stick of celery.)
Prepare the vegetables and slice evenly. Melt the
margarine in a large heavy saucepan, add the vegetables
and stir gently for 10 minutes. Add the garlic, salt and pepper,
and stir well. Add the tomatoes, tomato purée and herbs, and
then stir in the stock and bring to the boil. Cover and simmer
gently for 30 minutes. Add the strained and rinsed cannellini
beans and the pasta, and cook for a further 15 to 20 minutes.
(Incidentally, dried haricot beans can be used instead of
cannellini beans, but using tinned pre-cooked beans is
quicker and easier.) Check the seasoning. Serve with grated
Edam cheese sprinkled over the top.

Serves 4: 180 calories per portion

Guacamole with crudités

2 tomatoes
½ small onion
2 ripe avocado pears
juice of a whole lemon
1 clove garlic (crushed)
2·5 ml (½ tspn) Worcestershire sauce
30 ml (2 tbspns) natural low-fat yoghurt
salt
freshly milled black pepper

Ingredients for the crudités
4 carrots
4 sticks celery

½ cucumber
1 green pepper
1 red pepper

Skin and chop the tomatoes. Grate the onion. Halve the
avocado pears, remove the stones, scoop out the flesh, and
mash with the lemon juice. Add the onion, tomatoes, garlic,
Worcestershire sauce and yoghurt. Mix until smooth and add
salt and pepper to taste. Place in serving dish.

Cut the vegetables into even matchstick-sized pieces.
Put the avocado mixture on a large plate and arrange the
vegetables around it. The strips of vegetable are used to dip
into the avocado mixture.

Serves 4: 100 calories per portion

Smoked mackerel pâté

225 g (8 oz) smoked mackerel, skinned and boned
55 g (2 oz) low-fat spread
juice of 1 lemon
freshly milled black pepper

Flake the flesh of the mackerel and place in a liquidizer or
food processor. Add the low-fat spread and lemon juice.
Process until smooth. Season. Place in a serving dish, cover
with cling film and chill. Serve with slices of wholemeal toast
and lemon wedges.

Serves 4: 140 calories per portion

Home-made low-calorie soups are an enormous boon to slimmers
because they can be very filling (and also very warming on a cold
winter's day!).

French onion soup

15 g (½ oz) polyunsaturated margarine
455 g (1 lb) onions
2 cloves garlic (crushed)
2·5 g (½ tspn) low-calorie granulated sweetener

850 ml (1½ pints) beef stock (see comment, p. 148)
freshly milled black pepper

Heat the margarine in a large saucepan. Slice the onions and
add to the margarine. Stir in the garlic, add the sweetener,
and cook over a low heat for 15 minutes until the onions
brown. Pour on the stock, bring to the boil, cover and simmer
gently for 30 minutes. Season to taste and sprinkle with
parsley.

Serves 4: 50 calories per portion

Grapefruit cocktail

1 grapefruit
1 orange
10 ml (2 tspns) low-calorie granulated sweetener
2 sprigs of mint

Cut the grapefruit in half, remove the segments, and place
each skin in a bowl. Peel the orange and divide it into
segments. Mix the segments of the two fruits together with the
sweetener until the sweetener has dissolved. Place the fruit
in the grapefruit skins and top with the sprigs of mint. Serve
chilled.

Serves 2: 60 calories per portion

Leeks à la Grecque

340 g (12 oz) leeks
3 tomatoes
1 clove garlic, crushed
15 ml (1 tbspn) polyunsaturated oil
juice of ½ lemon
salt
freshly milled black pepper
chopped parsley to garnish

Wash the leeks and cut into 2 to 3 cm (one inch) lengths. Skin
and chop the tomatoes. Put the leeks, tomatoes and other
ingredients into a pan and season to taste. Simmer gently for

20 minutes, then allow to cool. To serve, transfer to a serving dish and serve cold garnished with parsley.

Serves 4: 60 calories per portion

MAIN COURSES

Beef and wine casserole

455 g (1 lb) braising steak
2 onions
2 carrots
2 sticks celery
115 g (4 oz) mushrooms
2 cloves garlic, crushed
2·5 g (½ tspn) dried thyme
285 ml (½ pint) red wine
1 beef stock cube

Cut off all the visible fat from the meat. Cut the meat into chunky cubes and fry gently in a non-stick pan until brown. Meanwhile, chop all the vegetables and then add to the browned meat and sauté for about 5 minutes. Add the rest of the ingredients, stir well, and cover with a close-fitting lid. Place in the middle of a pre-heated oven, gas mark 3, 325°F (160°C), for 3½ hours.

Serves 4: 265 calories per portion

Chicken Maryland

4 chicken breasts
1 egg white
salt
freshly milled black pepper
55 g (2 oz) wholemeal breadcrumbs
4 bananas
55 ml (4 tbspns) orange juice

Skin the chicken breasts. Lightly beat the egg white and season with salt and pepper. Dip the chicken breasts in the egg white, then coat evenly with the breadcrumbs. Place the chicken breasts in a baking dish and bake in a pre-heated oven, gas mark 5, 375°F (190°C), for 45 to 60 minutes. 15 minutes before the end of the cooking time, peel the bananas and slice in half lengthwise. Dip the bananas in the orange juice and place around the chicken breasts in the oven.

Serves 4: 270 calories per portion

Veal in breadcrumbs

1 egg white
1 escalope of veal
30 g (1 oz) breadcrumbs
30 g (1 oz) polyunsaturated margarine
¼ lemon (to garnish)

Beat the egg white and dip the veal in it. Then dip the veal in the breadcrumbs, pressing the breadcrumbs firmly to the meat. Leave to set in a fridge for about an hour. Melt the margarine in a non-stick frying pan and fry the veal for about 5 minutes on each side. Garnish with lemon.

Serves 1: 255 calories

Roast meats

Roasted meats, without any added fats, so beloved in many cookery books, are easy to cook and are an excellent way of preparing meat because some of the fat is lost during the cooking. Roast beef, served with horseradish sauce and wholemeal Yorkshire pudding (see recipe below), is delicious.

Wholemeal Yorkshire pudding

115 g (4 oz) wholemeal flour
1 egg
285 ml (½ pint) skimmed milk (or 30 ml (2 tbspns) skimmed milk powder dissolved in 285 ml (½ pint) water)

15 g (½ oz) polyunsaturated margarine
salt (just a pinch)

Make the batter *either* by sieving the flour and salt into a
mixing bowl, adding the milk and egg and mixing to a smooth
batter *or* by mixing the same ingredients in a blender or food
mixer. Melt the margarine in a Yorkshire pudding tin in a
pre-heated oven, gas mark 7, 425°F (220°C), until the fat is hot.
Pour in the batter and cook for about 30 minutes.

Serves 6: 110 calories per portion

When roasting lamb choose leg rather than shoulder as it is
much leaner. Serve whenever possible with *fresh* mint sauce.

Roast lamb with garlic

2 cloves garlic
1360 g (3 lb) leg of lamb
5 g (1 tspn) rosemary
5 g (1 tspn) thyme
4 medium potatoes
3 onions
salt
freshly milled black pepper
285 ml (½ pint) meat stock (see comment, p. 148)

Cut the garlic into small slivers and, using a sharp knife, make
slits at 2-inch intervals all over the leg and insert the garlic
into the slits. Rub the herbs all over the leg and place it in a
roasting tin in a pre-heated oven, gas mark 8, 450°F (230°C),
for 30 minutes. Meanwhile peel and slice the onions and
potatoes, place in a large bowl, and season with salt and
pepper. Layer the potatoes and onions around the leg in the
tin, pour the hot stock over the vegetables, and return the tin
to the oven for a further 1½ hours, reducing the temperature if
the potatoes seem to be browning too quickly. Serve with

fresh mint sauce. This is a delicious way of serving a joint without gravy.

Serves 4: 300 calories (assumes 115 g, 4 oz, portions of lean meat)

Minced meat dishes

When using minced beef in recipes, try to buy good quality mince that is not too fatty. Alternatively buy chuck steak or stewing steak, cut off all the visible fat, and mince the meat yourself.

The following recipe is a less fattening variation on classical Spaghetti Bolognese. The calorie savings come from using only 5 ml (one teaspoon) instead of 15 ml (one tablespoon) of oil and avoiding flour to thicken the sauce.

Spaghetti Bolognese

5 ml (1 tspn) olive oil
1 small onion
1 clove garlic, crushed
225 g (8 oz) lean minced beef
225 g (8 oz) tinned tomatoes
30 ml (2 tbspns) tomato purée
30 ml (2 tbspns) red wine
5 g (1 tspn) dried basil
salt
freshly milled black pepper
285 g (10 oz) spaghetti

Heat the oil in a heavy-based saucepan, add the onion (finely chopped) and garlic, and fry gently for 5 minutes. Turn up the heat and add the meat to brown it, stirring it all the time with a wooden spoon. Pour off any excess fat. Add the tomatoes, tomato purée, wine, basil, salt and pepper, give it all a good stir, turn the heat down, cover and simmer gently for 30 minutes. If you want a thicker sauce take the lid off and allow to bubble gently for a further 20 minutes.

Meanwhile, in a large open pan, bring some salted water to the boil and add the spaghetti. Boil the spaghetti for 20

minutes until it is tender but not soggy, and then drain it.
Serve the spaghetti with the Bolognese sauce poured over it.

Serves 4: 430 calories per portion

Chicken

Chicken is a good friend to healthy slimmers because it is relatively low in cholesterol and saturated fats and also in calories, especially when roasted, grilled or poached. It is a good food to experiment with to create new dishes. (Incidentally, chicken skin is extremely calorific, so do try to avoid eating it!)

Lemon chicken

4 chicken breasts
55 ml (4 tbspns) fresh lemon juice
rind of one lemon (grated)
30 ml (2 tbspns) polyunsaturated oil
2 cloves garlic (crushed)
salt
freshly milled black pepper

Place the chicken breasts in a greased shallow baking dish. Mix the lemon juice, rind, oil and garlic together. Lightly sprinkle the chicken pieces with a little salt and pepper. Pour the lemon mixture evenly over the chicken. Cover and bake in an oven, gas mark 4, 350°F (180°C), for 45 minutes, basting occasionally. Remove the cover and cook for a further 15 minutes to allow the chicken to brown slightly. Before serving, remove the chicken skin and sprinkle with chopped parsley.

Serves 4: 210 calories per portion

Fish

White fish is low in calories provided that it is not fried or served in rich creamy sauces, but grilled or baked with just a little lemon juice. For example, a 170 g (6 oz) portion of plaice fried in batter has 475 calories, whereas the same portion grilled contains less than 160 calories.

Fillet of sole with mushrooms

1 onion
225 g (8 oz) mushrooms
15 g (½ oz) polyunsaturated margarine
4 (115 g, 4 oz each) fillets of sole
15 g (1 tbspn) chopped parsley
salt
freshly milled black pepper
55 ml (4 tbspns) lemon juice

Peel and chop the onion, slice the mushrooms and fry gently in the margarine until lightly browned. Place the fillets in a heavy-based casserole, cover with the onion and mushroom mixture. Sprinkle with the parsley, salt and pepper and pour over the lemon juice. Cover and simmer for 25 minutes.

Serves 4: 145 calories per portion

Vegetarian main courses

Vegetable lasagne

170 g (6 oz) wholewheat lasagne
225 g (8 oz) celery, chopped
1 large onion, chopped
115 g (4 oz) green pepper, chopped
15 ml (1 tbspn) olive oil
1 clove garlic, crushed
115 g (4 oz) mushrooms, sliced
395 g (14 oz) tinned tomatoes
15 ml (1 tbspn) tomato purée
5 g (1 tspn) mixed herbs
175 ml (6 oz) red wine*
salt
freshly milled black pepper

---

* If you prefer to omit the wine, substitute vegetable stock.

Sauce
30 g (1 oz) wholemeal flour
350 ml (¾ pint) skimmed milk
25 g (1 oz) polyunsaturated margarine suitable for cooking
140 g (5 oz) cheese, grated

Cook the lasagne as instructed on the packet. Meanwhile, fry
the celery, onion and pepper lightly in the oil for about 5
minutes, add the garlic and mushrooms, and stir for a further 5
minutes. Add the tomatoes, tomato purée and mixed herbs.
Stir in the wine and season with salt and pepper. Allow to
simmer gently for about 10 minutes.

Make the sauce by whisking together the flour, milk and
margarine in a saucepan until smooth. Thicken the sauce by
bringing it gently to the boil, season with salt and pepper.
Add 115 g (4 oz) of the grated cheese and remove from the
heat.

Arrange a layer of vegetable mixture on the bottom of a
greased, oblong, ovenproof dish, cover with a layer of
lasagne, followed by a little cheese sauce. Place another
layer of vegetable mixture, followed by another layer of
lasagne, and pour the rest of the cheese sauce over the top.
Sprinkle with the rest of the cheese and bake in a pre-heated
oven, gas mark 5, 375°F (190°C), for about 40 minutes until the
surface is golden. Serve with a salad of your choice.

Serves 4: 455 calories per portion

Mushroom and onion bake

30 g (1 oz) polyunsaturated margarine
1 medium onion, chopped
225 g (8 oz) mushrooms, chopped
2 large eggs
275 ml (½ pint) skimmed milk
salt
freshly milled black pepper

(Similar to a quiche but without the pastry.)

Heat the margarine in a saucepan, add the onion and soften for a few minutes. Add the mushrooms and cook for about 20 minutes, stirring occasionally. Arrange evenly in the bottom of a greased dish.

Whisk the eggs and milk together, and season with salt and pepper. Pour the eggs over the mushrooms and bake in a pre-heated oven, gas mark 4, 350°F (180°C), for about 35 minutes, until the centre is set. (If you like you can add a few courgettes or tomatoes or any vegetable you have before you add the eggs.) Serve immediately.

Serves 2: 250 calories per portion

PUDDINGS

Ideally it is best not to have a sweet tooth so that you can avoid puddings which tend to be pretty calorific. However, for those who find a sweet ending to a meal a 'must', here are a few suggestions.

Peach Melba

275 ml (½ pint) low-fat natural yoghurt
2·5 ml (½ tspn) liquid sweetener
1 egg white
2·5 ml (½ tspn) vanilla essence
55 g (2 oz) raspberries
1 peach

Blend together the yoghurt and sweetener and chill in the freezer. Whisk the egg white. Turn the yoghurt mixture into a bowl, add the vanilla essence and egg white, and freeze until firm. Sieve the raspberries to make a smooth purée and blend together with the sweetener to taste. Scoop out the ice-cream, serve with the purée, and decorate with slices of peach.

Serves 2: 100 calories per portion

Fruit salad

2 oranges
2 apples
1 banana
1 pear
¼ melon
115 g (4 oz) strawberries
55 g (2 oz) grapes (preferably seedless)
55 ml (4 tbspns) fresh orange juice
liquid or granulated sweetener to taste

Peel, slice and chop the fruit, as appropriate, and mix
together. Add the orange juice to stop the fruit from
discolouring and also to provide necessary fluid. Taste and
sweeten as you wish.

Serves 4: 75 calories per portion

Lemon jelly with banana

1 packet of lemon jelly
juice of 1 lemon
1 banana

Make the jelly as instructed on the packet. Stir in the lemon
juice and allow to cool. Slice the banana thinly. Pour a layer of
jelly, half an inch to an inch deep, into a mould and allow to
set. Arrange the banana slices over this and then carefully
pour the remaining jelly mixture over the banana. Allow to set.

Serves 4: 30 calories per portion

Fruit Pavlova or slimmers' meringue

3 large egg whites
5 ml (1 tspn) cream of tartar
45 g (3 tbspns) skimmed milk powder
30 g (2 tbspns) granulated sweetener
1 410 g (14½ oz) tin of fruit salad in unsweetened syrup *or*
   home-made fruit salad (see above)
6 sprigs mint

Whisk the egg whites, add the cream of tartar, and continue
whisking until the mixture stiffens and peaks form. Add the
skimmed milk powder and sweetener, and continue whisking
until peaks form again. On a sheet of non-stick paper, draw a
circle round an 8-inch plate. Place on a baking sheet, and
spread (or pipe) the mixture smoothly in the circle. Cook in a
pre-heated oven, gas mark 1, 275°F (140°C) for one hour.
Cool, then loosen carefully with a palette knife and place on a
serving dish. Drain the fruit salad and pile on top of the
meringue, and top with the sprigs of mint.

Serves 4: 115 calories per portion

Chocolate soufflé

430 ml (¾ pint) skimmed milk
30 g (2 tbspns) cornflour
30 g (2 tbspns) cocoa powder
10 ml (2 tspns) liquid sweetener
55 ml (4 extra tbspns) skimmed milk
3 egg whites
5 ml (1 tspn) vanilla essence

Heat the 430 ml (¾ pint) of skimmed milk. Carefully mix the
cornflour, cocoa powder and sweetener with the 55 ml (4
tbspns) of cold skimmed milk to form a smooth paste. Gently
add to the hot milk and cook, stirring constantly, until the
mixture thickens. Remove from the heat and allow to cool.
Whip the egg whites with the vanilla essence until stiff, and
fold into the cold chocolate mixture. Spoon the mixture into a
serving dish. Serve chilled and decorated with a little grated
chocolate.

Serves 4: 90 calories per portion

The following dish is one of my wife's and my favourites and is always a great hit at dinner parties.

Crêpes Suzette

115 g (4 oz) plain flour (or part plain and part wholemeal)
3 tbspns granulated sweetener
285 ml (½ pint) skimmed milk (or 2 tbspns skimmed milk powder dissolved in 285 ml (½ pint) water)
1 egg white
juice and finely grated grated rind of 2 medium oranges
30 ml (2 tbspns) Cointreau or Grand Marnier
15 ml (1 tbspn) cooking brandy

Make the batter *either* by sieving the flour and half the sweetener into a mixing bowl, adding the milk and egg and mixing it to a smooth batter, *or* by mixing the same ingredients in a blender or food mixer. Using a non-stick frying pan, cook wafer-thin pancakes, using a *minute* amount of polyunsaturated oil to grease the pan. If you use a 7-inch pan, you should get about 9 pancakes. Stack them using grease-proof paper to prevent them sticking together.

Next, make the Suzette sauce by mixing together the rest of the sweetener, orange juice and rind, and orange liqueur. Spread the sauce evenly over each pancake and roll each pancake up. Place the pancakes side by side in a flameproof dish and place in a pre-heated oven, gas mark 7, 425°F (220°C), for 10 minutes.

To serve, bring to the table, pour the brandy from a well-heated ladle over the pancakes, and ignite (having first switched off the room lights!). Spoon the liqueur and sauce over the pancakes, and serve.

Serves 4 to 6 (depending on greed!): 70 calories in each pancake

Apple and lemon compote

455 g (1 lb) cooking apples
30 ml (2 tbspns) lemon juice
2 cloves
285 ml (½ pint) water
liquid sweetener to taste

Peel and core the apples and place in a pan with the lemon juice, water and cloves. Cook gently until the fruit is soft, and then remove the cloves. Serve hot or cold.

Serves 4: 50 calories per portion

SAUCES

Home-made low-calorie vinaigrette dressing

40 ml (3 tbspns) wine vinegar
15 ml (1 tbspn) polyunsaturated oil
5 ml (1 tspn) Worcestershire sauce
5 g dry mustard
2 drops liquid sweetener

Put the ingredients into a screw-top jar and shake well.

60 calories per 30 ml (1 oz)

There are two recipes for home-made low-calorie low-cholesterol mayonnaise. The first takes longer to make, but is lower in calories than the second. Which you use depends on individual taste and how lazy you are feeling.

Home-made low-calorie low-cholesterol mayonnaise (1)

285 ml (½ pint) skimmed milk
15 g (½ oz) cornflour
7·5 g (1½ tspn) dry mustard
5 g (1 tspn) paprika
12 drops liquid sweetener

2·5 g (½ tspn) salt
100 ml (6 tbspns) polyunsaturated oil
100 ml (6 tbspns) vinegar or lemon juice

Mix the milk and cornflour together in a saucepan to make a
paste, and cook until thickened. Place the paste in a bowl,
add the mustard, paprika, sweetener and salt, and beat the
ingredients until smooth. Gradually add the oil and vinegar
(or lemon juice), beating all the time, until the mixture is
blended.

60 calories per 30 ml (1 oz)

Home-made low-calorie low-cholesterol mayonnaise (2)

285 ml (½ pint) skimmed milk
225 ml (8 oz) polyunsaturated oil
40 ml (3 tbspns) vinegar or lemon juice
7·5 g (1½ tspn) dry mustard
5 g (1 tspn) paprika
12 drops liquid sweetener
2·5 g (½ tspn) salt

Blend all the ingredients together in a food processor or
blender into a smooth, thick mixture.

105 calories per 30 ml (1 oz)

Each of these mayonnaises has only a fraction of the saturated fats
and cholesterol of an ordinary bought mayonnaise and only about a
quarter of the calories. If you feel that making your own mayonnaise is too much bother, you can use a commercial sunflower
(mayonnaise style) dressing which, though not quite so low in
calories, has a highly acceptable taste. Each 30 ml (1 oz) has about
150 calories and just over 2 g saturated fat.

How fattening is food?

Food is as fattening as the number of calories contained in it. The following list of calorie values (taken mainly from *The Composition of Foods* – the Medical Research Council's Special Report No. 297 by R. A. McCance and E. W. Widdowson, published by HM Stationery Office) is for foods as eaten unless otherwise shown. The figures are averages as individual samples can vary.

Calorie Value of Common Foods

	Average portion	Calories per portion
Meat, Poultry and Fish		
Bacon	55 g (2 oz)	360
gammon	55 g (2 oz)	252
Beef, sirloin, roast	55 g (2 oz)	218
(lean only)	55 g (2 oz)	128
hamburger, fried	85 g (3 oz)	312
stewed steak	85 g (3 oz)	164
corned beef	85 g (3 oz)	198
Chicken, boiled or roast (joint)	115 g (4 oz)	216
Duck, roast	115 g (4 oz)	356
Ham, boiled, lean	55 g (2 oz)	124
Heart	85 g (3 oz)	81
Kidneys, stewed	85 g (3 oz)	135
Lamb or mutton, roast	85 g (3 oz)	249
chop, grilled	85 g (3 oz)	324
roast shoulder	85 g (3 oz)	300

	Average portion	Calories per portion
Liver (ox), fried	115 g (4 oz)	342
Luncheon meat	115 g (4 oz)	380
Pork, medium fat leg, roast	85 g (3 oz)	270
cutlets, fried	85 g (3 oz)	465
chops, grilled, lean	85 g (3 oz)	276
Sausages, beef, fried	85 g (3 oz)	243
black	55 g (2 oz)	162
breakfast	55 g (2 oz)	164
pork, fried	115 g (4 oz)	372
Steak and kidney pie	170 g (6 oz)	540
Sweetbreads	115 g (4 oz)	205
Toad-in-the-hole	170 g (6 oz)	492
Tongue	115 g (4 oz)	335
Tripe	115 g (4 oz)	115
Turkey, roast	55 g (2 oz)	112
Veal, roast	85 g (3 oz)	198

Sea Food

	Average portion	Calories per portion
Caviar	30 g (1 oz)	75
Cockles (without shells)	55 g (2 oz)	28
Cod, steamed	225 g (8 oz)	184
fried	225 g (8 oz)	464
Crab meat	85 g (3 oz)	108
Eel, stewed	85 g (3 oz)	318
Fish fingers (three)	85 g (3 oz)	145
Fish paste	20 g (¾ oz)	36
Haddock, steamed	170 g (6 oz)	168
Herring, in vinegar	170 g (6 oz)	324
Kedgeree	115 g (4 oz)	172
Lobster (½ lobster)	85 g (3 oz)	102
Mackerel, boiled	170 g (6 oz)	234
Oysters, raw (without shells) 12	115 g (4 oz)	56
Pilchards, tinned	115 g (4 oz)	216
Plaice, boiled	170 g (6 oz)	84
Prawns, boiled	115 g (4 oz)	120
Salmon, steamed	115 g (4 oz)	216
tinned	85 g (3 oz)	117

	Average portion	Calories per portion
Sardines, solids + oils	55 g (2 oz)	168
solids only	55 g (2 oz)	120
Shrimps, boiled	115 g (4 oz)	128
Sole, steamed	115 g (4 oz)	96
Trout, steamed	115 g (4 oz)	120
Tuna	85 g (3 oz)	220

Fruit

	Average portion	Calories per portion
Apples	one	60
Apricots, fresh	115 g (4 oz)	32
stewed without sugar	115 g (4 oz)	24
tinned, sweetened	115 g (4 oz)	120
dried, raw	55 g (2 oz)	104
cooked without sugar	115 g (4 oz)	68
Avocado pears (half)	85 g (3 oz)	75
Bananas (one)	115 g (4 oz)	88
Blackberries, fresh	115 g (4 oz)	32
Cherries, fresh	115 g (4 oz)	44
Cranberry sauce	15 g (½ oz)	30
Fruit cocktail, canned in syrup	115 g (4 oz)	108
Gooseberries, fresh ripe	115 g (4 oz)	40
Grapes, fresh (about 18)	85 g (3 oz)	51
Grapefruit, fresh (half)	115 g (4 oz)	12
(juice)	140 ml (5 fl. oz)	55
Lemon juice	30 ml (1 fl. oz)	2
Melons	170 g (6 oz)	24–42
Olives, green, in brine (four)	30 g (1 oz)	24
Oranges, fresh (one)	170 g (6 oz)	60
Orange juice	115 ml (4 fl. oz)	44
Peaches, fresh (one)	115 g (4 oz)	44
tinned, sweetened	115 g (4 oz)	100
Pears, fresh (one)	140 g (5 oz)	45
tinned, sweetened	115 g (4 oz)	88
Pineapple, fresh	115 g (4 oz)	52
tinned, sweetened	115 g (4 oz)	88
Plums, fresh	55 g (2 oz)	20
tinned, sweetened	115 g (4 oz)	88

	Average portion	Calories per portion
Prunes, stewed without sugar	115 g (4 oz)	76
Raisins, dried	30 g (1 oz)	70
Raspberries, fresh or stewed without sugar	115 g (4 oz)	28
Rhubarb, fresh raw	115 g (4 oz)	8
Strawberries, fresh	115 g (4 oz)	28
Sultanas	30 g (1 oz)	71

Vegetables

	Average portion	Calories per portion
Asparagus, fresh (8 spears)	115 g (4 oz)	20
tinned	115 g (4 oz)	12
Beans, baked	115 g (4 oz)	104
broad	115 g (4 oz)	48
french or runner	115 g (4 oz)	8
haricot, boiled	115 g (4 oz)	100
Beetroot, boiled	55 g (2 oz)	26
Broccoli, fresh	115 g (4 oz)	16
Brussels sprouts	85 g (3 oz)	15
Cabbage, fresh boiled	115 g (4 oz)	8
Carrots, fresh	85 g (3 oz)	18
tinned	85 g (3 oz)	15
Cauliflower, fresh boiled	115 g (4 oz)	12
Celery, stalk raw	85 g (3 oz)	9
Corn, sweet, fresh boiled	115 g (4 oz)	96
Cucumbers, fresh	55 g (2 oz)	6
Leeks, leaves	115 g (4 oz)	28
Lentils, dried	45 g (1½ oz)	104
Lettuce	5 g (¼ oz)	1
Marrow	170 g (6 oz)	12
Mushrooms	55 g (2 oz)	4
Onions, fresh boiled	115 g (4 oz)	16
fried	55 g (2 oz)	202
Parsnips, fresh	115 g (4 oz)	64
Peas, fresh	115 g (4 oz)	56
Peppers, raw	115 g (4 oz)	30
Potatoes, chips	115 g (4 oz)	272
boiled	115 g (4 oz)	92

	Average portion	Calories per portion
crisps	30 g (1 oz)	159
roast	115 g (4 oz)	140
Radishes, fresh	55 g (2 oz)	8
Spinach, fresh or tinned	115 g (4 oz)	28
Swedes, boiled	115 g (4 oz)	20
Tomatoes, fresh	115 g (4 oz)	16
Tomato juice	140 ml (5 fl. oz)	25
Turnips, fresh and greens	85 g (3 oz)	9
Watercress	30 g (1 oz)	4

Nuts (without shells)

Almonds (about 14)	30 g (1 oz)	170
Brazils (about 8)	30 g (1 oz)	180
Cashews, roast	30 g (1 oz)	170
Chestnuts, raw (about 7)	30 g (1 oz)	49
Coconuts, fresh	30 g (1 oz)	104
desiccated	30 g (1 oz)	178
Hazelnuts	30 g (1 oz)	190
Peanuts, roasted (about 18)	30 g (1 oz)	166
Walnuts (about 12)	30 g (1 oz)	156

Cereals and their products

Biscuits, plain	55 g (2 oz)	226
sweet	55 g (2 oz)	316
Bread (large loaf)	1 slice	65–72
lightly buttered	1 slice	135
fried	1 slice	185
Cake, fruit	55 g (2 oz)	220/282
Cornflakes, Rice Krispies, Shredded Wheat, Weetabix	30 g (1 oz)	100/104
Cornflour	30 g (1 oz)	100
Custard, made with milk and sugar	115 g (4 oz)	128
Energen rolls, Figgerolls	55 g (2 oz)	36
Flour, raw	30 g (1 oz)	100
Macaroni, boiled	30 g (1 oz)	32
Milk puddings, various	225 g (8 oz)	320
Oatmeal, raw	30 g (1 oz)	115

	Average portion	Calories per portion
Pastry, shortcrust	55 g (2 oz)	280
Rice, polished raw	30 g (1 oz)	102
Ryvita	2 pieces	68
Spaghetti, canned, with tomato sauce	115 g (4 oz)	70
Suet pudding	170 g (6 oz)	630
Trifle	170 g (6 oz)	258
Yorkshire pudding	115 g (4 oz)	252

Dairy products

	Average portion	Calories per portion
Butter (per slice)	5 g (¼ oz)	55
Cheese, Camembert	45 g (1½ oz)	132
Cheddar	45 g (1½ oz)	180
Cottage	45 g (1½ oz)	45
Cream	45 g (1½ oz)	348
Danish Blue	45 g (1½ oz)	154
Dutch	45 g (1½ oz)	116
Edam	45 g (1½ oz)	132
Gorgonzola	45 g (1½ oz)	155
Processed	45 g (1½ oz)	135
Stilton	45 g (1½ oz)	202
Cream, single	30 ml (1 fl. oz)	62
double	30 ml (1 fl. oz)	131
Eggs, whole (one)	55 g (2 oz)	92
fried (one)	55 g (2 oz)	136
Margarine (per slice)	5 g (¼ oz)	55
Milk, pasteurized (1 cup)	170 ml (6 fl. oz)	114
evaporated	30 g (1 oz)	41
condensed, sweetened	15 g (½ oz)	50
dried, skimmed (reconstituted)	170 ml (6 fl. oz)	60
Yoghurt (plain), low fat	140 ml (5 fl. oz)	75
(flavoured)	140 ml (5 fl. oz)	120

Fats

	Average portion	Calories per portion
Lard and suet	5 g (¼ oz)	65
Mayonnaise	15 g (½ oz)	103
Peanut butter (per slice)	5 g (¼ oz)	43

	Average portion	*Calories per portion*
Sauces and Condiments		
Bread sauce	30 g (1 oz)	32
Brown sauce	25 g (⅔ oz)	20
Cheese sauce	30 g (1 oz)	52
Olive oil	15 g (½ oz)	132
Salad cream	30 g (1 oz)	110
Salad dressing (French)	15 g (½ oz)	60
Tomato ketchup	25 g (⅔ oz)	18
White sauce	30 g (1 oz)	41
Worcester sauce	15 g (½ oz)	12
Garlic		
Mustard		
Pepper	negligible calories	
Salt		
Vinegar		
Soups		
Home-made	very variable	
Packet or tinned, thick	285 g (10 oz)	90–200
clear	285 g (10 oz)	40–65
Confectionery, puddings, sweets and sugar		
Apple pie	115 g (4 oz)	216
Blancmange	115 g (4 oz)	136
Boiled sweets (about 2)	55 g (2 oz)	46
Chocolate, milk	55 g (2 oz)	334
plain	55 g (2 oz)	310
Chocolates, assorted (about 2)	30 g (1 oz)	66
Custard	85 g (3 oz)	99
Fruit gums	30 g (1 oz)	49
Golden syrup	15 g (½ oz)	42
Honey	30 g (1 oz)	82
Ice cream	55 g (2 oz)	112
Jams (per slice)	15 g (½ oz)	37
Jellies (as eaten)	85 g (3 oz)	69
Lemon curd (per slice)	15 g (½ oz)	43

	Average portion	Calories per portion
Marmalade (per slice)	15 g (½ oz)	37
Pancakes	55 g (2 oz)	170
Peppermints	30 g (1 oz)	110
Rice pudding	115 g (4 oz)	168
Suet pudding	115 g (4 oz)	400
Sugar	5 g (1 tsp)	30
Sweeteners, artificial	5 g (1 tsp)	0
Toffees	30 g (1 oz)	120
Treacle	30 g (1 oz)	73
Trifle	115 g (4 oz)	172

Beverages (non-alcoholic)

Orange, lemon, grapefruit squashes	55 ml (2 fl. oz)	72/78
Low-calorie squashes	55 ml (2 fl. oz)	3
Bitter lemon, can	330 ml (11½ fl. oz)	110
Bovril (diluted)	140 ml (5 fl. oz)	5
Chocolate, drinking (made with milk)	140 ml (5 fl. oz)	175
Coffee (half milk, 2 tsp sugar)	140 ml (5 fl. oz)	115
Coca-cola, can	330 ml (11½ fl. oz)	125
Cocoa powder	5 g (½ oz)	64
Coffee (no milk or sugar)	170 ml (6 fl. oz)	6
Horlicks	15 g (½ oz)	56
Lucozade	170 ml (6 fl. oz)	114
Ovaltine powder	15 g (½ oz)	54
Oxo, 1 cube		15
Ribena	30 ml (1 fl. oz)	65
Tea (no milk or sugar)	170 ml (6 fl. oz)	6
Tonic water, can	330 ml (11½ fl. oz)	90
Slimline tonic water, can	330 ml (11½ fl. oz)	1
Other low-calorie carbonated drinks, can	330 ml (11½ fl. oz)	1

Alcohol

Beer, ale	285 ml (½ pt)	70–90
Stout	285 ml (½ pt)	100–110
Strong ale	285 ml (½ pt)	210
Brandy	30 ml (1 fl. oz)	73

	Average portion	Calories per portion
Champagne	115 ml (4 fl. oz)	84
Cider, dry	285 ml (½ pt)	100
sweet	285 ml (½ pt)	120
vintage	285 ml (½ pt)	280
Gin	30 ml (1 fl. oz)	63
Lager	285 ml (½ pt)	60
Lager, diabetic	285 ml (½ pt)	110
Liqueurs (most)	30 ml (1 fl. oz)	74
Port	55 ml (2 fl. oz)	86–90
Rum	30 ml (1 fl. oz)	63
Shandy	285 ml (½ pt)	150
Sherry, dry	55 ml (2 fl. oz)	66
sweet	55 ml (2 fl. oz)	76
Whisky	30 ml (1 fl. oz)	63
Wines, white	115 ml (4 fl. oz)	84–104
red	115 ml (4 fl. oz)	72–80

Foods with no or negligible calories
Tea without milk, cream or sugar
Coffee without milk, cream or sugar
Plain water
Carbonated water
Mineral water
Low-calorie squashes
Low-calorie carbonated drinks
Artificial sweeteners
Salt
Pepper
Mustard
Garlic
Curry powder
Lemons and lemon juice
Vinegar

Appendix A
Maximum Desirable Weights for Adults
(irrespective of age)

Height without shoes		Weight from			to		
ft in	cm	st	lb	kg	st	lb	kg

MEN

5 3	160·0	9	2	58·1	10	10	68·0
5 4	162·6	9	5	59·4	11	0	69·9
5 5	165·1	9	9	61·2	11	4	71·7
5 6	167·6	9	13	63·0	11	9	73·9
5 7	170·2	10	3	64·9	12	0	76·2
5 8	172·7	10	7	66·7	12	4	78·0
5 9	175·3	10	12	68·9	12	8	79·8
5 10	177·8	11	2	70·8	12	13	82·1
5 11	180·3	11	6	72·6	13	4	84·4
6 0	182·9	11	10	74·4	13	9	86·6
6 1	185·4	12	1	76·7	14	0	88·9
6 2	188·0	12	5	78·5	14	5	91·2
6 3	190·5	12	9	80·3	14	10	93·4

WOMEN

4 11	149·9	7	10	49·0	9	3	58·5
5 0	152·4	7	11	49·4	9	6	59·9
5 1	154·9	8	2	51·7	9	9	61·2
5 2	157·5	8	5	53·1	9	13	63·0
5 3	160·0	8	8	54·4	10	3	64·9
5 4	162·6	8	12	56·2	10	7	66·7
5 5	165·1	9	2	58·1	10	11	68·5
5 6	167·6	9	6	59·9	11	1	70·3
5 7	170·2	9	10	61·7	11	5	72·1
5 8	172·7	10	1	64·0	11	10	74·4
5 9	175·3	10	5	65·8	12	1	76·7
5 10	177·8	10	9	67·6	12	7	79·4

(Adapted from the Metropolitan Life Insurance Company 1960 tables)
The weights include indoor clothes and shoes (without clothes and shoes subtract 10 lb or 4·7 kg for men and 6 lb or 2·7 kg for women).

Note on use of table of Maximum Desirable Weights:

The table shows the *range* of weights for each height. Some books and magazines indicate weights for different frame sizes – small, medium and large. The problem is that no reliable method has yet been devised to determine whether your frame is in fact small, medium or large. Various methods have been described using such criteria as wrist circumference and shoe size, but these are often inaccurate guides to frame size. The only way to decide which build you are is to look at yourself in a mirror (but not through rose-tinted spectacles!) and, perhaps with the help of your husband or wife or other relative or friend, make up your mind about it. You can then judge whereabouts in the range of weights you should fit. If, without clothes, you look broad-shouldered and muscular your weight should be around the upper end of the range; if you look narrow-shouldered and not muscular your weight should be around the lower end of the range for your height. Most people fit somewhere in the middle which is where to place yourself if in doubt.

Appendix B

Range of Heights and Weights – Boys

Age (yrs)	Height from ft in	to ft in	Height from cm	to cm	Weight from st lb	to st lb	Weight from kg	to kg
Birth	1 7½	1 11	50·2	57·8	5½	9½	2·5	4·4
¼	1 10½	2 1½	56·6	64·7	10	16½	4·7	7·4
½	2 1	2 4½	63·8	72·6	1 0	1 8	6·4	9·9
¾	2 2½	2 6½	67·9	77·4	1 2½	1 11	7·5	11·5
1	2 4	2 8	71·2	81·4	1 4½	1 13½	8·3	12·6
1¼	2 5	2 9½	74·0	84·7	1 5½	2 1½	8·9	13·5
1½	2 6	2 10½	76·5	87·8	1 6½	2 3½	9·4	14·3
1¾	2 7	2 11½	78·7	90·5	1 7½	2 5	9·8	14·9
2	2 8	3 0½	80·7	93·1	1 8½	2 6½	10·2	15·6
2½	2 9	3 2	83·5	96·9	1 10	2 9	10·9	16·9
3	2 10½	3 4	87·0	101·4	1 12	2 12	11·6	18·0
3½	2 11½	3 5½	90·4	105·7	1 13	3 0	12·3	19·2
4	3 1	3 7	93·5	109·7	2 1	3 3	13·0	20·4
4½	3 2	3 8½	96·5	113·5	2 2	3 6	13·7	21·8
5	3 3	3 10	99·4	117·2	2 4	3 9	14·4	23·2
5½	3 4½	3 11½	102·2	120·8	2 5	3 13	15·1	24·8
6	3 5½	4 1	104·9	124·3	2 7	4 2	15·9	26·5
6½	3 6½	4 2½	107·6	127·6	2 9	4 6	16·6	28·3
7	3 7½	4 3½	110·3	130·8	2 11	4 11	17·4	30·3
7½	3 8½	4 4½	112·9	133·9	2 12	5 1	18·2	32·3
8	3 9½	4 6	115·4	137·0	3 0	5 6	19·1	34·4
8½	3 10½	4 7	117·9	139·9	3 2	5 10	20·0	36·5
9	3 11½	4 8½	120·4	142·9	3 4	6 1	21·0	38·8
9½	4 0½	4 9½	122·8	145·8	3 6	6 6	21·9	41·0
10	4 1½	4 10½	125·1	148·5	3 8	6 11	23·0	43·3
10½	4 2	4 11½	127·2	151·4	3 11	7 4	24·0	46·3
11	4 3	5 1	129·4	154·4	3 13	7 11	24·9	49·3
11½	4 4	5 2	131·7	157·8	4 1	8 5	26·0	53·3
12	4 4½	5 3½	133·7	160·9	4 4	9 0	27·1	57·2
12½	4 5½	5 4½	136·3	164·4	4 6	9 8	28·1	61·0
13	4 6½	5 6	138·7	168·2	4 9	10 2	29·6	64·4

| Age | Height | | | Height | | Weight | | | Weight | |
| (yrs) | from | | to | from | to | from | | to | | from | to |
	ft in		ft in	cm	cm	st lb		st	lb	kg	kg
13½	4	7½	5 7½	141·5	172·0	4	13	10	9	31·2	67·8
14	4	9	5 9½	145·0	176·2	5	3	11	2	33·3	70·9
14½	4	10½	5 10½	148·4	179·6	5	9	11	8	36·0	73·7
15	5	0	6 0	152·3	182·4	6	2	11	13	39·0	75·9
15½	5	1	6 0½	155·9	184·3	6	10	12	2	42·7	77·5
16	5	2½	6 1	158·9	185·5	7	3	12	5	45·7	78·6
16½	5	3½	6 1½	160·7	186·2	7	6	12	7	47·5	79·5
17	5	3½	6 1½	161·7	186·8	7	9	12	8	48·6	80·2
18	5	4	6 1½	162·2	187·2	7	12	12	10	50·0	81·0
19	5	4	6 1½	162·2	187·2	7	13	12	12	50·4	81·6

Range of Heights and Weights – Girls

| Age | Height | | | Height | | Weight | | | Weight | |
| (yrs) | from | | to | from | to | from | | to | | from | to |
	ft in		ft in	cm	cm	st lb		st	lb	kg	kg
Birth	1	7½	1 10½	49·2	56·8		5½		9½	2·6	4·4
¼	1	9½	2 1	54·9	63·1		9½	1	1	4·4	6·9
½	2	0	2 3½	61·1	69·9		13	1	6	5·9	9·1
¾	2	2	2 5½	65·5	74·9	1	1½	1	9½	7·0	10·6
1	2	3	2 7	69·1	79·3	1	3	1	12	7·8	11·8
1¼	2	4½	2 8½	72·2	82·9	1	4½	2	0	8·3	12·7
1½	2	5½	2 10	74·9	86·2	1	5½	2	1½	8·9	13·5
1¾	2	6½	2 11	77·2	89·1	1	6½	2	3½	9·3	14·3
2	2	7½	3 0	79·4	91·8	1	7½	2	5	9·7	14·9
2½	2	8½	3 1½	82·2	95·6	1	9	2	8	10·5	16·3
3	2	9½	3 3½	85·7	100·2	1	11	2	11	11·4	17·6
3½	2	11	3 5	89·2	104·5	1	13	3	0	12·2	18·9
4	3	0½	3 6½	92·3	108·5	2	1	3	3	13·1	20·3
4½	3	1½	3 8½	95·4	112·4	2	2	3	6	13·8	21·8
5	3	2½	3 9½	98·2	116·1	2	4	3	9	14·6	23·3
5½	3	4	3 11	101·0	119·6	2	6	3	13	15·4	25·0
6	3	5	4 0½	103·8	123·1	2	8	4	3	16·2	26·8
6½	3	6	4 2	106·4	126·4	2	9	4	7	17·0	28·5
7	3	7	4 3	109·1	129·6	2	11	4	11	17·8	30·6
7½	3	8	4 4½	111·7	132·8	2	13	5	2	18·6	32·6

Range of Heights and Weights – Girls (contd.)

Age (yrs)	Height from ft in	to ft in	Height from cm	to cm	Weight from st lb	to st lb	Weight from kg	to kg
8	3 9	4 5½	114·2	135·8	3 1	5 7	19·4	35·0
8½	3 10	4 6½	116·7	138·8	3 2	5 13	20·2	37·7
9	3 11	4 8	119·3	141·9	3 4	6 5	21·0	40·6
9½	4 0	4 9	121·9	145·0	3 6	6 12	21·8	43·8
10	4 1	4 10½	124·5	148·3	3 8	7 7	22·7	47·7
10½	4 2	5 0	127·1	151·8	3 10	8 2	23·6	51·7
11	4 3	5 1½	129·5	155·8	3 12	8 11	24·7	55·7
11½	4 4	5 3	132·0	160·1	4 2	9 5	26·2	59·6
12	4 5	5 4½	135·0	163·6	4 5	9 13	27·8	63·3
12½	4 6½	5 5½	139·0	166·1	4 9	10 6	29·7	66·5
13	4 8	5 6½	142·6	168·5	5 0	10 12	32·0	69·3
13½	4 9	5 7	144·4	170·3	5 6	11 2	34·5	71·1
14	4 10	5 7½	147·6	171·6	5 11	11 5	37·0	72·3
14½	4 11	5 8	149·4	172·7	6 3	11 7	39·5	73·2
15	4 11	5 8	150·3	173·2	6 8	11 8	41·7	73·7
15½	4 11½	5 8½	150·6	173·4	6 12	11 9	43·5	74·1
16	4 11½	5 8½	150·9	173·5	7 0	11 10	44·6	74·5
17	4 11½	5 8½	150·9	173·5	7 3	11 11	45·7	74·9
18	4 11½	5 8½	150·9	173·5	7 3	11 11	46·0	75·0
19	4 11½	5 8½	150·9	173·5	7 3	11 11	46·1	75·1

Tables adapted with kind permission of the authors and editor from: Tanner J. M., Whitehouse R. H. and Takaishi M. Standards from birth to maturity for height, weight, height velocity and weight velocity: British Children, 1965, part 2, *Arch. Dis. Childh.* (1966), vol. 41, pages 613ff. (The original tables express heights and weights in centimetres and kilograms. For convenience I have added their equivalents in feet and inches and stones and pounds.)

The heights and weights indicated cover ninety-four per cent of children, that is, three per cent of children will be shorter and lighter and three per cent will be taller and heavier than the range shown. When using these tables you should remember that a short child should have a weight at the lower end of the range; similarly a tall child will have a weight at the upper end of the range.

Index

FOR THE BEST IN PAPERBACKS, LOOK FOR THE (🐧)

In every corner of the world, on every subject under the sun, Penguin represents quality and variety – the very best in publishing today.

For complete information about books available from Penguin – including Pelicans, Puffins, Peregrines and Penguin Classics – and how to order them, write to us at the appropriate address below. Please note that for copyright reasons the selection of books varies from country to country.

In the United Kingdom: For a complete list of books available from Penguin in the U.K., please write to *Dept E.P., Penguin Books Ltd, Harmondsworth, Middlesex, UB7 0DA*

In the United States: For a complete list of books available from Penguin in the U.S., please write to *Dept BA, Penguin, 299 Murray Hill Parkway, East Rutherford, New Jersey 07073*

In Canada: For a complete list of books available from Penguin in Canada, please write to *Penguin Books Canada Ltd, 2801 John Street, Markham, Ontario L3R 1B4*

In Australia: For a complete list of books available from Penguin in Australia, please write to the *Marketing Department, Penguin Books Australia Ltd, P.O. Box 257, Ringwood, Victoria 3134*

In New Zealand: For a complete list of books available from Penguin in New Zealand, please write to the *Marketing Department, Penguin Books (NZ) Ltd, Private Bag, Takapuna, Auckland 9*

In India: For a complete list of books available from Penguin, please write to *Penguin Overseas Ltd, 706 Eros Apartments, 56 Nehru Place, New Delhi, 110019*

In Holland: For a complete list of books available from Penguin in Holland, please write to *Penguin Books Nederland B.V., Postbus 195, NL–1380AD Weesp, Netherlands*

In Germany: For a complete list of books available from Penguin, please write to *Penguin Books Ltd, Friedrichstrasse 10 – 12, D–6000 Frankfurt Main 1, Federal Republic of Germany*

In Spain: For a complete list of books available from Penguin in Spain, please write to *Longman Penguin España, Calle San Nicolas 15, E–28013 Madrid, Spain*

FOR THE BEST IN PAPERBACKS, LOOK FOR THE

PENGUIN HEALTH

Audrey Eyton's F-Plus   Audrey Eyton

'Your short-cut to the most sensational diet of the century' – *Daily Express*

Caring Well for an Older Person   Muir Gray and Heather McKenzie

Wide-ranging and practical, with a list of useful addresses and contacts, this book will prove invaluable for anyone professionally concerned with the elderly or with an elderly relative to care for.

Baby and Child   Penelope Leach

A beautifully illustrated and comprehensive handbook on the first five years of life. 'It stands head and shoulders above anything else available at the moment' – Mary Kenny in the *Spectator*

Woman's Experience of Sex   Sheila Kitzinger

Fully illustrated with photographs and line drawings, this book explores the riches of women's sexuality at every stage of life. 'A book which any mother could confidently pass on to her daughter – and her partner too' – *Sunday Times*

Food Additives   Erik Millstone

Eat, drink and be worried? Erik Millstone's hard-hitting book contains powerful evidence about the massive risks being taken with the health of consumers. It takes the lid off the food we eat and takes the lid off the food industry.

Pregnancy and Diet   Rachel Holme

It *is* possible to eat well and healthily when pregnant while avoiding excessive calories; this book, with suggested foods, a sample diet-plan of menus and advice on nutrition, shows how.

FOR THE BEST IN PAPERBACKS, LOOK FOR THE

PENGUIN HEALTH

Medicines: A Guide for Everybody   Peter Parish

This sixth edition of a comprehensive survey of all the medicines available over the counter or on prescription offers clear guidance for the ordinary reader as well as invaluable information for those involved in health care.

Pregnancy and Childbirth   Sheila Kitzinger

A complete and up-to-date guide to physical and emotional preparation for pregnancy – a must for all prospective parents.

The Penguin Encyclopaedia of Nutrition   John Yudkin

This book cuts through all the myths about food and diets to present the real facts clearly and simply. 'Everyone should buy one' – *Nutrition News and Notes*

The Parents' A to Z   Penelope Leach

For anyone with a child of 6 months, 6 years or 16 years, this guide to all the little problems involved in their health, growth and happiness will prove reassuring and helpful.

Jane Fonda's Workout Book

Help yourself to better looks, superb fitness and a whole new approach to health and beauty with this world-famous and fully illustrated programme of diet and exercise advice.

Alternative Medicine   Andrew Stanway

Dr Stanway provides an objective and practical guide to thirty-two alternative forms of therapy – from Acupuncture and the Alexander Technique to Macrobiotics and Yoga.

FOR THE BEST IN PAPERBACKS, LOOK FOR THE

PENGUIN HEALTH

A Complete Guide to Therapy   Joel Kovel

The options open to anyone seeking psychiatric help are both numerous and confusing. Dr Kovel cuts through the many myths and misunderstandings surrounding today's therapy and explores the pros and cons of various types of therapies.

Pregnancy   Dr Jonathan Scher and Carol Dix

Containing the most up-to-date information on pregnancy – the effects of stress, sexual intercourse, drugs, diet, late maternity and genetic disorders – this book is an invaluable and reassuring guide for prospective parents.

Yoga   Ernest Wood

'It has been asked whether in yoga there is something for everybody. The answer is "yes" ' – Ernest Wood.

Depression   Ross Mitchell

Depression is one of the most common contemporary problems. But what exactly do we mean by the term? In this invaluable book Ross Mitchell looks at depression as a mood, as an experience, as an attitude to life and as an illness.

Vogue Natural Health and Beauty   Bronwen Meredith

Health foods, yoga, spas, recipes, natural remedies and beauty preparations are all included in this superb, fully illustrated guide and companion to the bestselling *Vogue Body and Beauty Book*.

Care of the Dying   Richard Lamerton

It is never true that 'nothing more can be done' for the dying. This book shows us how to face death without pain, with humanity, with dignity and in peace.

FOR THE BEST IN PAPERBACKS, LOOK FOR THE

PENGUIN HEALTH

The Prime of Your Life   Dr Miriam Stoppard

The first comprehensive, fully illustrated guide to healthy living for people aged fifty and beyond, by top medical writer and media personality, Dr Miriam Stoppard.

A Good Start   Louise Graham

Factual and practical, full of tips on providing a healthy and balanced diet for young children, *A Good Start* is essential reading for all parents.

How to Get Off Drugs   Ira Mothner and Alan Weitz

This book is a vital contribution towards combating drug addiction in Britain in the eighties. For drug abusers, their families and their friends.

The Royal Canadian Airforce XBX Plan for Physical Fitness for Men and The Royal Canadian Airforce XBX Plan for Physical Fitness for Women

Get fit and stay fit with minimum fuss and maximum efficiency, using these short, carefully devised exercises.

Pregnancy and Childbirth   Sheila Kitzinger

A complete and up-to-date guide to physical and emotional preparation for pregnancy – a must for prospective parents.

Naturebirth   Danaë Brook

A pioneering work which includes suggestions on diet and health, exercises and many tips on the 'natural' way to prepare for giving birth in a joyful relaxed way.

FOR THE BEST IN PAPERBACKS, LOOK FOR THE

GARDENING IN PENGUINS

The Adventurous Gardener   Christopher Lloyd

Prejudiced, delightful and always stimulating, Christopher Lloyd's book is essential reading for everyone who loves gardening. 'Get it and enjoy it' – *Financial Times*

The Magic Garden   Shirley Conran

The gardening book for the absolute beginner. 'Whether you have a window box, a patio, an acre or a cabbage patch . . . you will enjoy this' – *Daily Express*

The Cottage Garden   Anne Scott-James

'Her history is neatly and simply laid out; well-stocked with attractive illustrations' – *The Times*. 'The garden book I have most enjoyed reading in the last few years' – *Observer*

Growing Fruit   Mary Spiller

From blossom to harvest, through planting, pruning, picking and storing, in a small or large garden, plot or pot, here is an illustrated step-by-step guide to growing fruit of all kinds.

The Illustrated Garden Planter   Diana Saville

How to choose plants for your garden – to cover a wall, creep between paving, provide colour in summer – and to plan for collective effect or to overcome a difficult site. 650 plants are illustrated, in all over 900 described.

Organic Gardening   Lawrence D. Hills

The classic manual on growing fruit and vegetables without using artificial or harmful fertilizers. 'Enormous value . . . enthusiastic writing and off-beat tips' – *Daily Mail*

FOR THE BEST IN PAPERBACKS, LOOK FOR THE

GARDENING IN PENGUINS

The Penguin Book of Basic Gardening   Alan Gemmell

From the perfect lawn to the flourishing vegetable patch: what to grow, when to grow and how to grow it. Given the garden, a beginner can begin on the day he buys this book with its all-the-year-round Gardener's Calendar.

The Pip Book   Keith Mossman

All you need is a pip and patience . . . 'The perfect present for the young enthusiast, *The Pip Book* should ensure that even the most reluctant avocado puts down roots and sends up shoots' – *The Times*

The Town Gardener's Companion   Felicity Bryan

The definitive book for gardeners restricted by the dimensions of their gardens but unrestrained by their enthusiasm. 'A fertile source of ideas for turning a cat-ridden concrete backyard into a jungle of soothing green' – *Sunday Times*

Water Gardening   Philip Swindells

A comprehensive guide to the pleasures and uses of expanses of water, however great or small in the garden. Includes advice on aquatic and marginal plants and the management of ornamental fish.

Beat Garden Pests and Diseases   Stefan Buczacki

An invaluable book, covering all types of plants, from seedlings to root vegetables . . . there is even a section on the special problems of greenhouses.

The Englishman's Garden   Alvide Lees-Milne and Rosemary Verey

An entrancing guided tour through thirty-two of the most beautiful individual gardens in England. Each garden is lovingly described by its owner. Lavishly illustrated.

FOR THE BEST IN PAPERBACKS, LOOK FOR THE

GARDENING IN PENGUINS

A History of British Gardening   Miles Hadfield

The great classic of gardening history. 'One of the most interesting, stimulating and comprehensive books to have come my way. It should be on every gardener's bookshelf . . . a remarkable book' – Cyril Connolly in the *Sunday Times*.

Roses for English Gardens   Gertrude Jekyll and Edward Mawley

Illustrated with beautiful photographs, this book demonstrates the nearly limitless possibilities for planting the best-loved flower of all – between walls, on pergolas, along wood posts, on verandas, and on trees.

Labour-Saving Gardening   Tom Wright

At last, a guide to make sure that you get maximum pleasure from your garden – with the least effort and just a little forethought and planning. Every aspect of gardening is investigated – all to save your most precious commodities: your energy and your time.

Gardens of a Golden Afternoon   Jane Brown

'A Lutyens house with a Jekyll garden' was an Edwardian catch-phrase denoting excellence, something fabulous in both scale and detail. Together they created over 100 gardens, and in this magnificent book Jane Brown tells the story of their unusual and abundantly creative partnership.

Window Boxes and Pots   Martyn Rix

Patio, balcony or windowsill – all can be transformed into an eye-catching delight with this wonderfully informative guide. Whether you settle for lobelia cascading from a hanging basket or geraniums of white, soft pink and cosy scarlet, you can be sure that Martyn Rix will tell you all you need to know.

FOR THE BEST IN PAPERBACKS, LOOK FOR THE

QUIZZES, GAMES AND PUZZLES

The Book Quiz Book   Joseph Connolly

Who was literature's performing flea . . .? Who wrote 'Live Now, Pay
Later . . .'.? Keats and Cartland, Balzac and Braine, Coleridge conun-
drums, Eliot enigmas, Tolstoy teasers . . . all in this brilliant quiz book.
You'll be on the shelf without it.

The Ultimate Trivia Game Book   Maureen and Alan Hiron

If you are immersed in trivia, addicted to quiz games, endlessly nosey,
then this is the book for you: over 10,000 pieces of utterly dispensable
information!

Unscrupulous?   Albie Fiore

Do you and your friends have principles? *Unscrupulous?* will help you to
find out. A book of moral choices and decision-making that will turn
friends into enemies, marriages into divorces and provide hours and hours
of entertainment.

Plus four new trivia quiz books:
The Royalty Game
The TV Game
The Travel Game
The Pop Game

Crossword Books to baffle and bewilder

Eleven Penguin Books of The *Sun* Crossword
Eight Penguin Books of the *Sunday Times* Crossword
Seven Penguin Books of *The Times* Crossword
and
Four Jumbo Books of The *Sun* Crosswords

The First Penguin Book of *Daily Express* Crosswords
The Second Penguin Book of *Daily Express* Crosswords

Penguin Crossword Books – something for everyone, however much or
little time you have on your hands.